CANCER SECRETS

CANCER SECRETS

An Integrative Oncologist Reveals
How You Can Defeat Cancer Using the Best of
Modern Medicine and Alternative Therapies

Jonathan Stegall, MD

ALPHARETTA, GA 36605
7705512730

ISBN: 978-1-7323273-0-6

Interior design by booknook.biz

To my late mother, Dr. Susan Stegall,
who died unexpectedly during the writing of this book.
She was - and still is - my hero and inspiration.

TABLE OF CONTENTS

INTRODUCTION

There are few things scarier than hearing those three words: "You have cancer." Unlike any number of other terrible diseases, cancer is common, it is aggressive, and the treatments for it are often as bad as the disease itself. Despite how terrifying those three words are, there are thousands of people every day that hear them. Over 1.6 million people in the United States were estimated to have been diagnosed with cancer in 2016, and nearly 600,000 people in this country will die from the disease this year.

It is currently estimated that 1 out of every 3 people will be diagnosed with cancer at some point in their lifetime, and this number is quickly approaching 1 in 2. This grim statistic serves as a sobering reminder that none of us are free from the scourges of this deadly and terrifying disease; whether it is experiencing the disease personally, or watching friends, family, or loved ones fight for their lives against it, it is unlikely that anyone has remained unaffected by cancer's ravages. Unfortunately, many epidemiological studies confidently predict that cancer will soon surpass heart disease as the number one killer of Americans.

I became a physician because I wanted to help people, to "get into the trenches" with them, so to speak. As I grew up, I would learn that my passion is walking with people through some of their darkest times, taking care of them when they need it most. For me, that meant taking care of sick people. I became an integrative oncologist, however, because I felt a real connection with cancer patients.

What I began to realize after years of medical training and taking care of cancer patients was that something is missing in our understanding of cancer and how we treat it. After years of research, billions of dollars spent, and countless lives lost, those statistics are no better than they were when we started. They are, in fact, far worse. Something significant must change in how we approach cancer.

———————•———————•———————

I was not always sure that I wanted to be a cancer specialist. Many doctors begin dreaming of going to medical school while they are still in grade school, but that is not my story. Even though I was unsure of the course that my life would take, from the time I was a little boy, my parents told me I was here to do big things. I was born at 29 weeks, weighing a mere one pound and fourteen ounces. The doctors gave me a 50/50 chance of surviving. While I am certainly grateful that I did make it, I do not believe it was an accident or a random act of chance. God gives us all a purpose, and I firmly believe He led me to mine.

I grew up in Greenville, South Carolina, with my mother and father. My mom was a doctor, and even though it would be later in life before I decided that I wanted to study medicine, Mom would become an important influence on who I was to become, both as a person and a physician.

From an early age, I remember her taking me to the doctor for yearly checkups, which is usual for most kids. Any time I was sick, of course, I got the medicine that I needed. I also remember, even as a very young boy, my mother breaking up nutritional supplements and putting them into my food. She always had the family on a variety of supplements as I was growing up. The "supplement cabinet," however, was not something I saw at my friends' houses.

Today, we have evidence that taking certain nutritional supplements may provide a variety of benefits for our health. Indeed, our knowledge of diet, nutrition and how our lifestyle affects our well-being has greatly expanded in recent years, but this knowledge was not always commonplace or readily available. In the 1980s, there was far less information available on the efficacy and utility of vitamins, minerals, herbs, phytonutrients, and nutrition in general. Supplements were largely relegated to fringe groups of "health nuts," and most people simply were not interested in vitamins or supplements. Certainly, there was far less open-mindedness toward such things in the medical community. In many ways, that attitude remains today, despite mounting evidence that nutrition can play a profound role in health.

My mother was certainly ahead of the curve in that regard. Growing up, I experienced, firsthand, the blending of conventional medical wisdom— the kind my mother learned in her training—and the importance of nutrition, supplements, and healthy lifestyle. In retrospect, it was my mother's prescient, open-minded attitude toward natural health that influenced who I was to become as an integrative oncologist.

●———————————————————●

My first experience with cancer came when I was in the first grade. My maternal grandmother was diagnosed with a form of stomach cancer. I was very close with my grandma growing up, and in retrospect, watching her struggle with cancer would be profoundly influential on me.

It was my mom who would walk me through this experience. I remember her explaining to me in 5-year-old terms that Grandma had a tumor, or a "growth" in her stomach. Grandma would need to have some aggressive treatments, like chemotherapy and radiation. My mom explained that grandma might not feel good for a while; she might lose a lot of weight and she might even lose all of her hair. I remember when that happened, my mom bought Grandma a wig and also came home with one for me, albeit a multi-colored clown wig. I remember my grandma and me wearing our wigs together after she lost all of her hair.

My grandmother's cancer was advanced—stage 4—and her condition rapidly deteriorated. Toward the end, I remember being in the hospital with my mother, and her explaining to me that grandma was in a coma, and that she was not really aware of what was going on. Ultimately, my grandmother passed away, and, like many people, my first experience with cancer also became my first experience with death. I was five years old.

Looking back, losing my grandma to cancer influenced me in a variety of ways. Importantly, I was old enough to realize how bad cancer is and the toll it takes on a patient, even the seemingly healthiest ones; I watched firsthand as my grandmother went from a lively, animated, and happy person to someone who was sick a lot, despite maintaining a great attitude. I also saw how her death affected our family.

I would go on to attend Clemson University, not far from where I grew up. Like a lot of college kids, I still did not really know what I wanted to do with my life. I majored in business, because that seemed like a good thing to do at the time, still not realizing I was destined to become a doctor, much less an integrative oncologist. It was not until I was getting close to graduating that a few things would solidify my direction into medical school.

As I was going through college, my grandfather went into kidney failure. Kidney patients require quite a bit of care, including regular trips to a dialysis center. Throughout the process of helping my parents take care of my grandfather, I realized that I truly enjoyed helping people in this way. I enjoyed caring for people and being with them throughout the process of fighting illness.

This is what we do as doctors. We get into the trenches with our patients; their fight becomes our fight. This was my passion, walking with people through some of their darkest times. I felt like I could make a difference, even if only by being a friend and encourager to those that were sick. At this time, I knew God was calling me into medicine. Ultimately, the decision to pursue medicine was as much a spiritual decision as it was a career choice. Through watching my grandparents get ill, and having the opportunity to walk through that process with them, God had shown me my passion. I faithfully followed His direction.

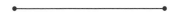

After college, I was accepted into Georgetown University to obtain my master's degree in physiology. This was not just any master's degree program, but rather, a special, one-of-a-kind program which consisted of a track in complementary and alternative medicine. Sponsored by a grant from the National Institutes of Health, my master's program included rigorous science courses as well as classes in alternative medicine. The program did not take a stance on alternative medicine, but instead, taught us how to approach research studies and clinical trials in an unbiased way so that we would have the tools necessary to form our own opinions and draw our own conclusions.

The summer following my master's degree, I completed a research internship at Harvard Medical School's Osher Center for Integrative Medicine. Here, I conducted research on the doctor-patient relationship, and its potential impact on treatment outcomes. Not surprisingly, I found that this sacred relationship between physician and patient plays a profound role.

Following my research internship, I went on to attend the Medical University of South Carolina. No one would say that medical training is an easy time in the life of any doctor; the stress, workload, and sheer volume of material for which you are responsible can fray the strongest of nerves, and this is before you ever set foot in a hospital. Medical training has a way of shaping who you become as a physician beyond just the training, itself. For me, there are two cases from my medical training which have stuck with me as especially influential, in terms of who I was to later become as an integrative oncologist.

The first case happened while I was still in medical school. The first two years of medical school are primarily classroom-based, with lectures and exams, similar to college courses—but much more intense! The second two years are primarily clinical training, during which time you work in hospitals and clinics in tandem with doctors who are treating patients.

In my third year of medical school, I was working at the Veterans Administration Hospital, which was one of the hospitals we rotated through as part of our clinical training. A patient who was around 60 years old presented to the hospital; he had been diagnosed with stage 4 stomach cancer that had metastasized to his liver. The tumors were big enough that they could be seen beneath the skin when he lifted his shirt up.

This patient had driven himself to the VA, which was a couple hours from where he lived. He was unmarried, and while I believe he had children, they were not particularly involved in his life. Any other family he had was estranged. The patient checked himself into the hospital for a couple of weeks to receive treatment for the tumors, fully expecting to drive himself back home a few weeks later.

Perhaps because he had so little by way of friends or family, I became attached to him and would regularly visit him after I would finish my clinical day in the hospital. On other instances, I would visit him on the weekend, even when I was not working. I felt like I could make a difference, at the very least by becoming his friend and providing emotional and spiritual support as he underwent treatment for cancer.

Unfortunately, his case took a turn for the worse, and he died while in the VA hospital. This was my first experience with death of one of my patients. I remember sitting in my apartment crying, replaying his case in my mind to see if there was something I had missed which could have saved his life. Of course, given his poor prognosis when he arrived, my exercise was an unproductive one clinically, but a necessary one for me personally.

The second case that sticks out happened during my postgraduate training at Yale. At this point, I had received my medical degree and was a doctor in training.

A young woman, approximately 30 years old, presented to the oncology unit of the hospital where I was working. She had been treated for cancer via chemotherapy and radiation 10 years earlier, and had been in remission, but the cancer had returned aggressively.

In contrast to the older man I had worked with in the VA hospital, this young lady had a strong, helpful, encouraging family as well as a close group of friends. They stood by her side as she underwent treatment for cancer the second time, this time with an even grimmer prognosis. A strong support system for cancer patients is important; it can be a powerful resource for those going through treatment, and has been shown to improve treatment outcomes.

Perhaps because we were so close in age, I felt a strong connection to her. This, I thought, could very easily be me. Like I did with the older gentleman at the VA hospital, I befriended the young woman I was caring for, frequently visiting her after I was done for the day. Even though she had a supportive group of friends and family, I felt like I could make a difference in her life, both medically and as an encourager.

(In the process of caring for this young woman, I met one of the nurses who was caring for her, who I would eventually fall in love with and marry—another important reason this case sticks out in my mind.)

When she was readmitted to the hospital for the last time, she was assigned to another group of doctors who would handle her case. I knew that she was in a lot of pain toward the end, and despite her requests for more pain medication, her attending doctors would not allow her more. Ultimately, there was nothing I could do for her medically, or even palliatively, because she was not my patient in the end. Going against her attending physicians would have resulted in the loss of my job and possibly my medical license as well. I felt helpless.

In spite of all the care and support, the young woman died.

Between these two cases, I saw a man with no support system who did not believe he was going to die, and a woman who knew she was close to the end who did have a great support system. Sadly, both ended up with the same outcome. I felt personal connections with both of these patients, and I felt that I could help them at the very least by supporting them as a friend through their treatment. However, in both cases, I felt limited by what I could offer them medically. I felt confident that there must be more that I could do for them, and it became my life's work to discern what that might be.

This is not to disparage cancer treatment as it stands, necessarily. We have made tremendous strides in cancer care since my grandma was diagnosed with stomach cancer in 1985. Regardless, progress in medicine happens slowly. The old joke is that progress is made one physician death at a time, in terms of the old guard moving on and a younger generation moving into positions of authority. Sadly however, even amongst my peers, I see very little open-mindedness when it comes to thinking outside the box.

In medicine today, our treatments for cancer are based primarily on large-scale, randomized, double-blind, placebo-controlled clinical trials, which constitute the barometer for what becomes standard of care. Anytime we talk about things outside of that standard of care, the question becomes, what is the evidence for it? That brings forth a significant dilemma: in order to have those huge, consistent, long-term studies, you have to have a significant amount of funding. But who is going to fund a study of an off-label use of an existing medication? Who is going to fund a supplement study? Who will pay for a clinical trial on a novel nutritional intervention?

What we are left with are a lot of smaller studies that often times will show tremendous promise, but are not the level of evidence that those who set the standard of care go by. However, it *is* enough for those of us who are more open-minded to take a closer look at how this might work clinically with other therapies we are using.

My cancer treatment philosophy is as follows: if we have a scientific basis for how a treatment might work, and we do not believe it will harm the patient, then we should be open-minded about using it. If a small study shows promise using a specific intervention, and the patients in that study had a good outcome, that is significant to me. Although more evidence is typically better than less evidence, I do not believe we should restrict ourselves to large-scale studies exclusively. We MUST have an open mind about trying new therapies, even if the evidence is not yet clear. I believe that the success I have had with patients is evidence of this. I truly believe we are on to something.

I realize that a small study is not enough to make certain treatments the standard of care, or to garner insurance coverage, but I do feel that I am often speaking a different language than my peers, who are generally only interested in what they are taught at certain conferences or read in certain journals. From their perspective, if they were not taught something, it must be irrelevant. I find this to be a dangerous position to take, because there is so much we do not yet know about cancer.

Many of my patients have seen - and even experienced - this attitude within the medical community, and like me, they are frustrated. Coupled with the fact that many feel rushed during the short period of time they do get to spend with their physician, many feel like their doctor does not listen to them. Many turn to independent research via the internet. The internet has proven to be a powerful tool, in terms of informing people about cancer and some of the more natural therapies that may be beneficial in the fight against this nasty disease. Largely, this has driven much of the interest in natural medicine, but the medical community has been slow to change its paradigm.

It is true that we know more now than ever before about how nutrition and natural therapies might provide real benefits for patients, but as much information as there is available on how these remedies can be used against cancer, there probably exists equally as much misinformation. Unfortunately, I have seen many patients take matters into their own hands and try to fight cancer exclusively with natural remedies based on unscientific information they have gotten from less-than-qualified sources. In my experience, this rarely ends well.

I practice truly integrative oncology, because I believe that the best approach to fighting cancer includes both conventional and so-called "alternative" therapies. The fact is, we need methods like chemotherapy and surgery; how we use those methods and what we do *in addition* to those methods is how my practice distinguishes itself from more mainstream oncology clinics, as well as clinics which focus only on alternative therapies.

●————————————————●

There are three things I hope to accomplish by writing this book.

First, I want to introduce integrative oncology as a valid medical specialty whose goal is to address the rise in cancer rates and high death rates associated with cancer. While we have made some dramatic strides since 1971 when President Nixon declared war on cancer, it is fair to say that we are still losing, despite the billions of dollars we have spent toward that end. Clearly, something is amiss. Integrative oncology seeks to pick up where conventional oncology, alone, has left off.

Let me be clear in saying that integrative oncology is not the same as alternative medicine or natural medicine. In my practice, we still recommend surgery, chemotherapy, and radiation when appropriate. These are valid medical practices with science to back them up. Unlike conventional oncology, however, I believe they are simply an incomplete tool set.

There are very few oncologists practicing integrative medicine, but it is a movement. The movement toward natural health has grown exponentially in popularity in recent years, and this has primarily been driven by public demand. I expect what we do in integrative oncology to become more mainstream in years to come, because what we are doing is helping people in a profound way. Ultimately, it is my desire for this book to introduce integrative oncology to a broader audience as a legitimate, science-based practice.

Secondly, I hope to inform people that they have a variety of tools available to them in their fight against cancer. Too many people feel afraid to talk to their oncologist about anything outside the scope of conventional therapies, out of fear of being ridiculed or even dismissed by their doctors. It is important that people understand that there is a wider palette of effective therapies with legitimate science behind them, in addition to just surgery, chemotherapy, and radiation. By broadening their horizons, I am confident that people will see that cancer treatment can be better tolerated and more effective.

This book is not a step-by-step guide on how to treat cancer, nor is it necessarily the guaranteed guide to preventing cancer. At no point in the book will you see the word "cure." There is far too much that we do not understand about this disease to make that kind of claim, and it is important to approach anyone who makes such claims with extreme caution and skepticism. Furthermore, if you do have cancer, it is not recommended that you implement any of the methods discussed in the book without the assistance of a trained integrative oncologist.

Lastly, it is my goal to instill hope. John 10:10 says, "The thief comes to steal, kill and destroy." Cancer, in the realest sense, is that thief physically realized. It comes to steal our health, kill our bodies, and destroy our hope. Understandably, a diagnosis of cancer often brings with it deep despair.

The second part of that verse is, however, far more important, when Jesus says, "I have come that they may have life and have it to the fullest." As a believer, my faith is in the greatest of Healers; it is my faith that brings me hope. Spiritual health is as important as physical health, and that is something we stress in my practice.

Ultimately, not all outcomes with cancer treatment are the same, but I believe hope is one of the most important gifts you can give to someone who has received a cancer diagnosis. I believe hope is vital to navigating the trials of treatment, and it can be a powerful healing tool as well. I know that what we are doing in my practice brings hope to many for healing, for longer life, and for better quality of life.

CHAPTER 1

Where We Are, and How We Got Here

"What we've got here is a failure to communicate."
– Captain in Cool Hand Luke

A Brief History of Cancer

Cancer is perhaps the most confounding, terrifying, and elusive disease known to man. It is characterized by unchecked, rapid division of cells. Often, cancer results in tumors that destroy organs and tissues. A more in-depth description of what cancer is—and what it is not—is covered in later chapters. Before we jump into the science, it is vital to understand cancer from a historical perspective.

We know more about cancer today than ever before, but as much as we do know about this terrible disease, there is likely far more we do not yet know about it. As it stands, cancer is an epidemic, quickly becoming the biggest killer of Americans, but it has not always been this way. To better understand where we are as a society in terms of cancer incidence, treatment, and outcomes, it might help to know a little bit about where we have been.

Cancer is a disease that has affected man and animals for millennia. The earliest evidence of cancer affecting humans comes from fossilized bone tissue. Cancer appears in the autopsies of mummies from ancient Egypt, and we know that our ancient ancestors were aware of the disease, even if they did not understand its scope. (1, 5)

It was the Egyptians who first described cancer in writing around 3000 BC. In the Edwin Smith papyrus, Egyptian physicians describe 8 cases of tumors or ulcers of the breast that were removed via cauterization using a tool known as the fire drill. The text goes on to say that for the tumors, "There is no treatment." (1, 2) While there was no treatment for the tumors available at the time, it is here that we see the origins of surgery as a treatment for cancer.

Later, it was the Greek physician, Hippocrates, who would use the words, *carcinos* and *carcinoma,* to describe cancer tumors. These are Greek words for crab, which likely refer to the spindling projections coming off of cancer cells. (1, 3, 5) It is known that the Greeks would surgically remove cancerous tumors, often with painful, disfiguring surgeries.

The Romans would eventually translate the Greek words, *carcinos* and *carcinoma,* to the Latin word for crab, or cancer. (1, 3)

The Renaissance and the Birth of Modern Medicine

Through the middle ages, our understanding of the human body progressed very slowly. Scientific inquiry was frowned upon, and procedures such as autopsies were not allowed, largely for religious reasons. Many of the accepted ideas about the cause of disease had not appreciably changed since the time of Hippocrates. For people in these times, this meant accepting antiquated disease theories dating back thousands of years.

The Greek humoral theory of disease was the pervasive philosophy during the middle ages. The humoral theory posited that health was attained when the four humors, or liquids found within the body, were in balance. These four liquids were blood, lymph, yellow bile, and black bile. Cancer, it was thought, formed when an excess of black bile accumulated in the body. (3, 4)

It would not be until the Renaissance swept through Europe that physicians would begin to learn enough about the human body to begin developing more modern theories about cancer. Renewed scientific curiosity and the development of the scientific method would lead to new understanding about how the human body worked and how disease developed and progressed. As discoveries were made and knowledge progressed, various theories about what cancer was and what caused it would develop.

One theory which emerged during the Renaissance was that cancer was actually an infectious disease. This theory was arrived at virtually simultaneously by two doctors in Holland in the 17th century. Doctors Zacutus Lusitani (1575-1642) and Nicholas Tulp (1593-1674) both independently observed members within the same households developing breast cancer. (4) Both deduced that cancer, like the flu or other infectious diseases, could be transmitted from person to person. Both doctors recommended that cancer patients be isolated so the disease would not spread. In retrospect, the doctors were likely among the first to notice a genetic link to cancer, even if they mistook it for an infectious disease. We now know that human cancers are not contagious, but this theory persisted through the 18th century.

During the 18th century, the lymph theory of cancer would emerge to replace the long-held, ancient Greek humoral theory of cancer. Stahl and Hoffman posited that cancer was made of decaying and fermenting lymph fluid in varying degrees of density, alkalinity, or acidity. (4) The famous Scottish surgeon, John Hunter (1728-1793), would become a proponent of this theory. John Hunter was the first physician to suggest that certain cancers might be cured by surgery. He would note that if the tumors had not spread into surrounding tissues, it would be appropriate to excise them. (4, 5)

Simultaneously in the 1700s, Giovanni Morgagni (1682-1771) would be the first physician to perform autopsies on the deceased with the intent of finding correlations between illness and pathological findings.

(4, 5) This would become standard practice (as it is today) and would be critical for developing our understanding not just of cancer pathology, but all disease pathology.

19th and 20th Century Discoveries—Discovering the Causes of Cancer

More theories would subsequently replace the lymph and infectious theories of cancer in the 19th century. In 1838, a German pathologist named Johannes Muller (1801-1858) would determine that cancer was made up of cells, not lymph. Muller believed, however, that cancer cells were derived from budding elements between tissues, or blastema. This became known as the blastema theory of cancer. (4, 5)

With the development of more powerful microscope technologies in the 19th century, the physician Rudolf Virchow (1821-1902)—a student of Johannes Muller— would greatly advance our understanding of the cellular pathology of cancer. (4, 5) The ability of pathologists to examine cancer tissue under the microscope provided insight into the damage the disease caused, allowed for more precise diagnosis, and gave pathologists the ability to inform surgeons if all cancerous tissue had been removed during surgery.

Virchow believed that cancer was the result of chronic irritation. Virchow is credited with determining that all cells—even cancer cells— are derived from other cells, which disproved Muller's blastema theory of cancer. Virchow's theory became known as the chronic irritation theory. However, he incorrectly assumed that cancer spread like a fluid throughout the body. (4, 5) It was the German physician Karl Thiersch (1822-1895) in 1860 who is credited with discovering that cancer metastasized through the spread of malignant cells. (4, 5)

In 1895, German physicist Wilhelm Roentgen (1845-1923) discovered X-rays, a discovery that revolutionized medicine. During the course of his experimentation, he realized that his newly-discovered rays could pass through human flesh, but metal, bones and denser tissue would block varying degrees of the ray. When cast upon film, Roentgen realized that he could create images of the bones and tissues within the human body. A lecture he delivered in 1896 electrified the medical community, and within months, X-ray machines were being used in the diagnosis of diseases, including cancer. (6, 7) Shortly thereafter, it was discovered in France that daily doses of radiation greatly improved cancer patients' chance of survival. Fairly soon after X-rays had been discovered and implemented as a diagnostic tool, radiation therapy became a treatment for cancer patients with some success. (6)

Unfortunately, the dangers associated with the use of radiation were poorly understood before it was adopted as a diagnostic tool and as a treatment protocol; in the years following, many of the early radiologists would develop leukemia as a result of radiation exposure. Through these unfortunate events, it was discovered that ionizing radiation could both cause and treat cancer. Later, we would discover that other forms of radiation, such as ultraviolet radiation from sunlight (UV rays), gamma rays, and radon (a radioactive gas) can also contribute to increasing the risk of developing cancer.

The 20th century would lead to more discoveries about what many of the causes of cancer were. In 1911, Peyton Rous discovered a type of cancer in chickens that would eventually be proven to have been caused by a virus. Rous would receive the Nobel Prize for his work in discovering what would become known as the Rous sarcoma virus. (8) Since then, scientists have discovered a variety of viruses, such as hepatitis B, hepatitis C, Epstein-Barr, HIV, and human papilloma virus that can all cause a variety of cancers in the human body.

In 1915, researchers Katsusaburo Yamagiwa and Koichi Ichikawa at Tokyo University induced cancer in rabbits by applying coal tar to their skin. This prompted research into other chemical agents that can cause cancer in humans. (8) Today, we are aware of hundreds of chemical compounds that increase the risk of cancer in humans.

The early 20th century revealed some of the key causes of cancer. In cases of radiation, viral carcinogens, and chemical carcinogens, we realized that cancer had very clear environmental causes. The precise mechanism behind how those environmental factors caused cancer, however, had yet to be discovered.

Discovering DNA

In 1962, James Watson and Francis Crick were awarded the Nobel Prize for discovering the chemical structure of DNA, the basic coding material for the entire human body and all its functions. This discovery was pivotal for a number of reasons, but it was particularly key for how doctors, researchers, and scientists would view cancer moving forward. The discovery of DNA led to many answered questions about why cells would start dividing out of control.

DNA, it was discovered, was what ultimately gave commands to all cells; when sections of DNA, known as genes, would become damaged (known as a mutation), cells would divide out of control, leading to cancer. While it was known that radiation, certain chemicals, and viruses could lead to cancer, the mechanism behind how those carcinogens led to cancer could now be understood; these carcinogens, or cancer causing agents, all had the ability to damage our DNA. Furthermore, since every individual's DNA is inherited from their parents, it was realized that we could receive "bad" genes that predisposed us to cancer. In other words, DNA offered an explanation as to why cancer seemed to run in families.

The Growing Epidemic and the War on Cancer

Lifetime Risk of Death from Cancer

While our knowledge of cancer would grow exponentially in the 20th century, another terrifying trend was developing; cancer was quickly becoming the largest killer of people in the developed world.

Studies done in recent years have brought this trend into sharper focus. In 2012, The New England Journal of Medicine released a report entitled, *The Burden of Disease and the Changing Task of Medicine*. In this report, the doctors who authored the paper cited the major causes of death per 100,000 people in the year 1900. Infectious disease was the leading cause of death in the year 1900, and accounted for around 580 deaths per 100,000 people. (9) The second leading cause of death in the year 1900 was heart disease, which accounted for 137 deaths per 100,000 people. Cancer was responsible for claiming the lives of 64 people out of every 100,000.

Recall that in the year 1900, our understanding of cancer was very limited. X-rays had been discovered only 5 years before, and our knowledge of what caused cancer and how to treat it was still in its infancy.

The New England Journal of Medicine report chronicled the causes of death up until 2010. By the 1970s, the risk of death from cancer had increased to 162 out of 100,000 deaths, over two and a half times what the cancer death rate was in 1900. Cancer was now the second leading cause of death, behind heart disease.

By this point, the United States government had taken notice. In spite of all the advancements that had been made in medicine, it was clear that something needed to be done to address the issue of cancer. In 1971, President Nixon declared war on cancer, vowing to find a cure for the disease. He signed into law The National Cancer Act, pledging billions of dollars over the course of several years to fight the disease and establishing the National Cancer Institute. (10)

Now we had a "war" on cancer, with the government funneling billions of tax payer dollars into research and a search for a cure. Despite this enormous effort, the 2012 New England Journal of Medicine report stated that in 2010, the risk of death due to cancer was nearly 186 out 100,000, tripling from the rate in 1900.

Ultimately, after forty years and billions of dollars spent to wage war against cancer, the average outcome of cancer treatment had largely remained the same, if not worse since the 1970s.

Lifetime Risk of Developing Cancer

Obviously, for more people to be dying from cancer, there must be more people who are developing cancer. To this point, most of these statistics have been in reference to American populations, but a 2015 paper published in the British Journal of Cancer sought to compare risk of developing cancer today to the risk historically.

The paper compared the lifetime risk of two groups of men and women for developing cancer; the first group was born in 1930, the second in 1960. The study discovered that women born in 1930 had a 36.7% lifetime chance of developing cancer. By 1960, the risk was 47.5%. For men born in 1960, the risk increased to 53.5%, up from 38.5% for men born in 1930. (11)The paper ultimately concluded that for all adults under 65 years old, the risk for developing cancer is now greater than 50%.

Many argue that these statistics are largely skewed by a variety of factors: Many posit that we are finding cancer today because of better diagnostic tools, or because people are living longer, leading to a higher risk of developing the disease. Many cite that the death rate at birth is lower than it has ever been, which would arguably skew data, making it appear as though cancer incidence has increased.

The question is, accounting for all factors, have cancer rates still increased? Some studies suggest that they have. A study published in 2017 in the Journal of the National Cancer Institute indicates that people born after 1990 have double the chance of developing colon cancer as a young adult, and quadruple the risk of developing rectal cancer. (12) Though this is one study, it is likely as more information becomes available that we will see similar trends.

Regardless, as it stands, in spite of the billions spent in both private and public funds fighting this disease, it remains one of the top killers of people in the developed world.

The Standards of Care and Their Origins

As it stands today, there are three primary standards of care when it comes to cancer treatment: chemotherapy, radiation therapy, and surgery. If you are diagnosed with cancer, it is highly likely that you will be recommended a combination of some or all of these therapies. There are, however, other therapies within the standards of care that have become more mainstream, including immunotherapy and hormone therapy. Each standard of care has specific uses and a rich body of research and evidence to support its use.

Surgery

Surgery has been used to treat cancer since antiquity and is the oldest method used for treating cancer. Obviously, surgical techniques have come quite far since the first primitive surgeries in ancient times. While ancient people's methods might have been primitive, their intuition was far from it; it was well known that simply removing cancerous tissue via surgery did not amount to a cure. The second century physician Galen, who was considered the authority on cancer treatment for over a thousand years, considered a patient incurable upon a diagnosis of cancer. (5, 13) This attitude has remained into the 21st century—even when patients survive, they are considered in remission, never fully cured.

Surgery in ancient times was primitive and often fraught with complications, but it did take place. It was not until the 19th and 20th centuries that significant advancements in surgical procedures would be developed. In the 1890s, a professor of surgery at Johns Hopkins named William S. Halstead developed the radical mastectomy for cases of breast cancer, although the concept can be traced as far back as the 1700s, with the German physician Lorenz Heister. (13) The radical mastectomy would remain the standard practice for breast cancer patients up until the 1970s. In fact, for many cancers found in limbs, the standard practice was simply amputation.

Modern technology has allowed surgery to progress to the point of being minimally invasive and extremely precise. Imaging technology such as ultrasound, CT scans, MRI scans, and PET scans have eliminated much of the need for exploratory surgeries in cases of cancer; furthermore, they allow for much more precision when removing tumors.

Surgery often remains our first line of defense when it comes to cancer. However, the fact that cancer metastasizes, or spreads, remains one of the greatest limitations to surgery and necessitates that additional therapies typically be used in conjunction with surgery.

Chemotherapy

Chemotherapy is perhaps one of the most feared medical therapies in existence. Despite many advancements in chemotherapy that have mitigated the harsher side effects, at times the side effects are as bad as the disease itself. Chemotherapy works by killing rapidly growing cells, such as cancer cells.

Interest in chemotherapeutic agents began during World War II with studies on mustard gas. The US military was studying a variety of chemicals related to mustard gas with the intent of developing more effective chemical weapons. During the course of those studies, an agent called nitrogen mustard was discovered to be effective in fighting lymphoma. (14,15)

Following this discovery of nitrogen mustard, Sidney Farber of Harvard discovered that a compound called aminopterin caused remission in cases of acute leukemia in children. Aminopterin was a predecessor of methotrexate, a popular cancer drug still in use today. (14, 15) In the following years, much of the research into how to treat cancer would center around finding new chemotherapeutic agents.

Radiation Therapy

Radiation therapy has come a long way since Wilhelm Roentgen first gave his lecture on X-rays in 1896. Early machines used for administering radiation therapy were extremely crude in contrast to today's machines. Particularly, in the last 50 years, advancements in computer technology and the physics of radiation have given us more precise treatment with less collateral damage.

Today, conformal radiation therapy (CRT) and intensity-modulated radiation therapy (IMRT) deliver targeted doses of radiation that conform to the size of the tumor, which is mapped in 3D by computer imaging techniques.

The latest extension of radiation therapy is proton therapy, which uses protons instead of X-ray beams. Proton therapy is extremely targeted and largely eliminates collateral damage.

Immunotherapy

Immunotherapy constitutes a more modern approach to fighting cancer and is a blanket term for a variety of treatments. It is also called biological response modifier (BRM) therapy, biologic therapy, and biotherapy. Initially, the technology used in immunotherapy was used to find and diagnose tumors, but advancements in our understanding of these agents have made it possible to use them to actually destroy cancer cells. Immunotherapy was first approved in the 1990s for lymphoma and breast cancer, but is now routinely used in a variety of cancers.

Immunotherapy seeks to boost the body's natural cancer-fighting mechanisms. Many of the drugs given in this type of therapy are actually biologic agents that occur naturally in the body, such as interferons, interleukins and other cytokines.

Hormone Therapy

Certain cancers, such as cancers of the breast and prostate, are influenced by estrogen and testosterone, respectively. Hormone therapy in cancer treatment centers around the use of drugs to block these specific hormones to which certain cancers are sensitive. These drugs are also being studied for their use in preventing prostate and breast cancers.

Nothing Outside of the Standard

If a patient is diagnosed with any form of cancer, that patient will overwhelmingly be recommended any combination of the treatments within the standards of care. There is little else a patient will likely hear from an oncologist or their staff. These are the treatments they deal in, and there is little incentive for them to learn about anything outside of these treatments. Unfortunately, even when an oncologist is presented with a potential therapy or mode of treatment outside of the standard of care, it is likely he or she will show little interest in it. This is likely due to a combination of several factors, including a perceived lack of evidence for therapies outside the scope of practice, a lack of understanding and training in these therapies, and a genuine concern regarding the safety and compatibility of these therapies given in conjunction with the standard of care.

There have been dramatic strides in the fight against cancer, particularly in the last 50 years. The standards of care in use today have volumes of scientific literature to back their usage. Certainly, one would think that the outcomes in cancer care have equally grown in stride with our advancements in how we treat cancer. Particularly, if there is not an enormous, unilateral thrust to find anything outside of what we are currently using to treat cancer, what we have must certainly be working... Right?

Cancer Today: What Are We Missing?

In 2009, President Barack Obama detailed his mother's fight with ovarian cancer in an interview with Harper's Bazaar. In the interview, he said, "Now is the time to commit ourselves to waging the war on cancer as aggressive as the war cancer wages on us." His administration earmarked $1 billion of the $5 billion in federal medical research funding to search for genetic causes of cancer and new therapies.

Unfortunately, those words and figures sound a little too familiar. We have to ask ourselves, are we winning the war on cancer? Nearly 50 years after President Nixon first declared war on cancer, death rates remain virtually the same, if not worse, and a person's lifetime risk of developing the disease is higher than it has ever been before. Is more money funneled into the same channels going to fix the problem? Something is clearly missing.

Undoubtedly, the largest missing piece of the puzzle is our discussion about prevention. Despite increased public awareness regarding potential causes of cancer, cancer deaths continue to rise, and cancer is rapidly overtaking heart disease as the primary killer of Americans. The best advice we are given is typically, do not smoke. While this is good advice, it leaves quite a bit to be desired when it comes to cancer prevention. If we are going to address the huge rise in risk of developing cancer and the subsequent death rate associated with cancer, we have to begin with discussing the prevention of the disease.

There are two studies, specifically, that highlight how lacking our discussion on cancer prevention is, and what the implications are.

The first study was published in 2002 in the European Journal of Cancer Prevention. The researchers involved in the study examined the relationship between weight control, exercise, and incidence of cancer. Ultimately, the study concluded that between a quarter and one-third of a variety of cancers, including cancers of the colon, breast, endometrium, kidney, and esophagus, could be prevented with appropriate exercise and weight control. (16)

The second study, published in 2016 in the Journal of the American Medical Association, found similar results. The study concluded that maintaining a healthy weight and regular, weekly exercise reduced cancer risk by as much 40% in Caucasians. The study would also conclude that lifestyle modification could prevent nearly half of all cancer deaths. (17)

It is striking that up to 40% of cancers could be prevented, and roughly half of cancer deaths could be prevented, with improved lifestyle interventions. Yet, the average primary care physician spends very little time discussing specifics of healthy nutrition and exercise with patients. Moreover, once patients are diagnosed with cancer, the average oncologist tells patients that diet does not matter and that there is no evidence that nutrition makes a difference. Most never address the importance of exercise, and the discussion about weight is typically over a concern that patients not lose too much weight (ultimately leading to cachexia). Virtually none discuss the role of stress and the importance of stress management.

It is important to emphasize that a 40% reduction in cancer diagnoses would mean that nearly 800,000 people in the United States would not hear those dreaded words *every year*, yet this fact is largely glossed over. For the status quo to change, our discussion must begin with a serious and exhaustive discussion about cancer prevention.

Cancer Screening

As much as can be done in terms of preventing cancer, another shortcoming in the standard protocol for cancer prevention lies within our screening, or lack thereof. Unfortunately, as it stands, cancer is the second most prevalent disease, behind heart disease, but we come nowhere near the level of screening for cancer that we do for heart disease. Markers for heart disease are closely and routinely monitored if a patient regularly visits their primary care provider. One can even check their blood pressure at home with devices available at a pharmacy.

What has necessarily changed in terms of our screening for cancer, even as its prevalence has increased? If you are a woman, perhaps you will start getting Pap smears around age 21 or mammograms at age 40. If you are a man, you will likely start getting your prostate checked around age 40. At 50, hopefully, many will begin regular colonoscopies. Anything beyond these routine tests are unlikely.

We have the best chance for good treatment outcomes when cancer is diagnosed early; in order to diagnose cancer earlier, our current standards for screening must be improved upon.

Tunnel Vision in Cancer Treatment

The development of chemotherapy and immunotherapy, and the blossoming field of genetics have been critical to our efforts towards treating cancer, and understanding how it develops. Understandably, these developments have taken over much of the research in the medical community. This is, however, perhaps, to the detriment of the overall understanding of the disease and how best to treat it, or (ideally) prevent it. It is important to emphasize that these have been important developments that have been useful in saving lives; the problem lies within the fact that they have created a sort of tunnel vision in regard to where our researchers have looked for new breakthroughs in how to treat cancer.

Chemotherapy and Immunotherapy

Following the discovery of nitrogen mustard by the US army and the later discovery of aminopterin by Sidney Farber in the middle part of the last century, chemotherapy and the search for new chemotherapeutic agents created a new, primary focus for the medical and research community; the main thrust of research into cancer treatment has remained focused on drug development, which is dominated, today, by new immunotherapy drugs. Anything outside of this scope is largely ignored.

This is unfortunate, because the type of studies used to determine standards of care require a great deal of funding. The lion's share of that funding both from the private and public sector goes toward studies aimed at developing chemotherapy drugs and, more recently, immunotherapy drugs. What is left over is not typically enough to meaningfully fund anything in the realm of natural or alternative therapy. This is in addition to the fact that there is little incentive within the private drug sector to pour enormous amounts of funding into researching things like diet, high dose intravenous vitamin C, or other nutrients that cannot be patented.

The culminating result of these factors is that most oncologists never hear anything about the efficacy of treatments outside of what is published in major medical journals or taught at certain conferences. Usually, their interest in anything outside of information received via these avenues is lacking at best; often though, many oncologists are adamantly opposed to even entertaining the idea of trying treatments beyond what they learn about from the big medical journals or conferences.

This is not to disparage chemotherapy itself, which has saved many lives; or immunotherapy, which has shown promise for some types of cancers and is the major focus of research efforts today. We have seen dramatic improvements in these drugs' efficacy; however, they are far from perfect, and the challenge is finding out which drugs—and at what doses—are optimal for each patient.

The ultimate problem lies within the fact that there remains so much we do not know about cancer. The vast sums of money tied up in cancer research ultimately prohibit natural remedies from becoming more mainstream, despite the fact that these therapies are often both safe and effective. This very shortsighted approach is one reason why our outcomes in cancer treatment are as poor as they are.

It is in Your Genes

Similar to the discovery of cancer treatment drugs, the discovery of the role genetics plays in cancer has largely co-opted our search for the causes of cancer. Recall that before the discovery of DNA, many environmental causes of cancer had been (and were being) identified, including radiation, certain viruses, and chemical carcinogens. Largely, the discovery that damaged DNA leads to cancer halted our search into what damages DNA in the first place, and placed the blame on our genes themselves.

Some of these specific, "bad" genes have been identified, such as the BRCA1 and BRCA2 genes in breast cancer. Often, however, there are no unifying, specific genetic changes for specific types of cancer. In other words, just because a person has breast cancer or prostate cancer, we do not necessarily see specific abnormalities in genetics unique to those cancers.

Furthermore, the presence of genetic abnormalities associated with cancer does not necessarily guarantee that a person will develop cancer.

In recent years, genetic testing has become en vogue; part of that testing has centered around telling people what certain types of cancer for which they have a genetic predisposition. The problem is that those tests are very hard to interpret, and the FDA has since prohibited certain labs from offering these tests to the public.

Quite simply, the answer to cancer treatment does not lie in the identification and subsequent treatment of specific genetic abnormalities. Interestingly, even with all of the research that has been done on the genetic cause of cancer, our most aggressive estimations are that 6-8% of cancers are caused by genetics. (18) This leaves more than 90% that are not caused by genetics!

The belief that cancer is a genetic disease is rooted in the knowledge that damaged DNA causes cells to divide out of control, leading to cancer. The question becomes, however, what causes DNA to become damaged in the first place? The focus on genetics, specifically, has taken much of the attention away from this question; likely, we are mistaking the mechanism for the cause.

It is known that carcinogens and environmental agents play a role in the incidence of cancer. What is not typically addressed is the exponentially higher number of environmental contaminants we are regularly exposed to in modern society. Today, there are tens of thousands of chemicals in existence that were not around 100 years ago; these chemicals are in our air, water, food, drugs, cosmetics, clothes, furniture, and electronics, just to name a few. The overwhelming majority of these chemicals have not been studied as potential carcinogens. It is possible, if not very likely, that the genetic insults we are seeing that lead to cancer are the result of manmade carcinogens.

The knowledge that only a small fraction of cancers are purely genetic in origin, combined with the fact that our bodies are overwhelmed by an enormous number of unnatural chemicals that contaminate our everyday environment, certainly calls into question the idea that cancer is a genetic disease. This is something we will discuss more in chapter 2.

The Cost of Cancer

There are a variety of figures that estimate what cancer costs the U.S. economy. One study published in 2011 estimated the total cost of cancer care to be $124.57 billion in 2010, and that by 2020, that figure would grow to $157.77 billion. (19) The American Cancer Society estimated that the direct medical costs for cancer were $87.8 billion in 2014. (20) Another figure predicts that by 2020, cancer costs could soar to $175 billion per year. The National Institutes of Health estimated the total cost of cancer—including medical costs, mortality costs, and lost productivity—to be more than $216 billion. (21) Not only do these figures represent the astounding prevalence of cancer, but they also highlight the serious financial burden it places on our healthcare system.

As if receiving a diagnosis of cancer is not enough, cancer patients are often burdened by the crushing financial reality of the cost of treatment. According to the Agency for Healthcare Research Quality, the average cost per year for an individual's cancer treatment was $85,201. For those with insurance, out-of-pocket expenses could be as low as $3,644. (21) For those on medicare with no supplemental insurance, however, out-of-pocket expenses could be as high as $8,115. (22)

Parts of the high costs associated with cancer are due to the astronomically high prices of cancer drugs; a year's supply of some chemotherapy drugs is as high as $100,000. (21) The costs for immunotherapy drugs are even higher. These drugs can cost as much as $300,000 per patient per year. As one oncologist at Memorial Sloan Kettering Cancer Center in New York admitted, this is "about 4000 times the cost of gold." (23)

The high costs of fighting cancer have much to do with our attitude toward insurance; many assume that if they have insurance, all or most of their healthcare costs will be covered. This is, in part, why we have seen insurance rates skyrocket out of control for the past few decades. Drug companies, hospitals and other healthcare providers have little incentive to keep costs down when insurance covers much of the care. Furthermore, while healthcare providers may bill a certain amount for a drug or a procedure, insurance companies often only reimburse a percentage of what healthcare providers charge. This only leads healthcare providers to charge more for services; if healthcare providers charge more for services, insurance companies are forced to reimburse more.

Ultimately, however, the higher costs get passed on to the consumers. The rules outlined in ECON 101 apply here: there is no such thing as a free lunch. The huge sums of money that cancer care commands are coming from somewhere.

It is true that drug companies must invest enormous sums of cash in order to bring a drug to market, and this is part of the reason why the cost of many drugs are so high. Even when a chemotherapy drug costs merely cents to manufacture, that drug's availability is the result of many years and many hundreds of millions of dollars' worth of research.

It is worth noting, too, that the private sector stands to benefit very little from the discovery of natural interventions; diet, vitamins, or other "alternative" therapies simply are not their business, because those therapies can neither be patented, nor profited from in any meaningful way, at least compared to drugs. On the other hand, patentable chemotherapy or immunotherapy drugs can be very lucrative for the ones who develop them.

Costs not typically discussed are the emotional and spiritual costs associated with cancer. A diagnosis of cancer and the challenges of treatment can bring about feelings of anxiety, depression, and despair. Cancer, in the realest way, can cost an individual their quality of life, even with a good prognosis. We must realize that these are significant outcomes associated with cancer, but our standard protocol for cancer care does very little to address these very real results.

Interest in Natural Medicine: A Double-Edged Sword

Between the prevalence of cancer, the anxiety associated with the standard treatments for cancer, and the availability of information on the internet, many people have taken it upon themselves to educate themselves not only on what they can do if they are diagnosed, but also what they can do to prevent cancer from ever developing.

Often, cancer patients feel helpless, as if there is little they can do for themselves; they feel like they are at the mercy of their oncologist, their treatment, or chance. Today, however, cancer patients have access to more information than ever before via the internet, and in many ways this has become empowering.

A wealth of information exists on how to cope with a cancer diagnosis, and much of it is accessible online. The internet is also the primary source of information on therapies outside of the standards of care. One way patients can take control of their situation is by researching, and then incorporating, things like diet, nutritional supplements, and healthy lifestyle. For many, it allows them to feel like they are taking control over their health.

This, of course, becomes a double-edged sword. An abundance of good information *is* available for people to find. The internet also makes it easier for patients to connect with other cancer patients and to hear their success stories. Because of the abundance of information, however, this research can become overwhelming. Furthermore, even when patients do find potentially good information, many are not scientifically literate enough to accurately assess scientific studies or read the data involved. This unfortunately breeds much of the conspiracy-minded information on the internet. If a patient reads that a certain nutrient or plant derivative cures cancer, then certainly it must be "Big Pharma" or the government hiding something for economic reasons. Unfortunately, it is not so simple; just because a compound shows promise against cancer in vitro (or, in the lab), the implications are frequently much different in vivo (or, in the human body).

Often, too, there is conflicting information, or information that is difficult to incorporate into a regimen without the aid of an oncologist or other trained physician. Other times, there is just plain misinformation that gets popularized on the internet. Tragically, the availability of so much misinformation has led many people to take cancer treatment into their own hands by exclusively relying on natural therapies. While there are anecdotal accounts of people healing themselves in this way, they are often unsubstantiated at best. Typically, these cases end very poorly.

This is largely where integrative oncology can bridge the divide. The fact is, there are a variety of options cancer patients have when it comes to their treatment options. Many of these are within the standards of care, including chemotherapy, immunotherapy, radiation therapy, hormonal therapy, and surgery. Integrative oncology seeks to take the most promising aspects of therapies not necessarily within the standard of care and combine them with more conventional methods in an effective, scientific way which is personalized for each patient.

Ultimately, the interest in more natural ways of dealing with cancer is going to become a net-positive movement. Hopefully, a greater interest in treatments outside the standards of care will influence the ways in which we spend our research dollars, adding scientific validation to safe and effective methods of treating cancer in addition to the existing standards of care.

(1) "Early History of Cancer." American Cancer Society. N.p., n.d. Web. 26 July 2017.

(2) "History of breast cancer." Senology. N.p., n.d. Web. 26 July 2017.

(3) "Science Diction: The Origin Of The Word 'Cancer'." NPR. NPR, 22 Oct. 2010. Web. 26 July 2017.

(4) "Early Theories about Cancer Causes." American Cancer Society. N.p., n.d. Web. 26 July 2017.

(5) Olszewski MM. Concepts of Cancer from Antiquity to the Nineteenth Century. Univ Toronto Med J 2010; 87(3): 181-6.

(6) "Evolution of Cancer Treatments: Radiation." American Cancer Society. N.p., n.d. Web. 26 July 2017.

(7) "Wilhelm Conrad Röntgen - Biographical." Nobelprize.org. N.p., n.d. Web. 26 July 2017.

(8) "Development of Modern Knowledge about Cancer Causes." American Cancer Society. N.p., n.d. Web. 26 July 2017.

(9) Jones DS, Podolsky SH, Greene JA. The burden of disease and the changing task of medicine. N Engl J Med 2012; 366(25): 2333-8.

(10) "National Cancer Act of 1971." National Cancer Institute. N.p., n.d. Web. 29 June 2017.

(11) Ahmad AS, Ormiston-Smith N, Sasieni PD. Trends in the lifetime risk of developing cancer in Great Britain: comparison of risk for those born from 1930 to 1960. Br J Cancer 2015; 112(5): 943-7.

(12) "Study Finds Sharp Rise in Colon Cancer and Rectal Cancer Rates Among Young Adults." American Cancer Society. N.p., n.d. Web. 02 July 2017.

(13) "Evolution of Cancer Treatments: Surgery." American Cancer Society. N.p., n.d. Web. 26 July 2017.

(14) "Evolution of Cancer Treatments: Chemotherapy." American Cancer Society. N.p., n.d. Web. 26 July 2017.

(15) Mandal A. "History of Chemotherapy." News-Medical.net. N.p., 14 Jan. 2014. Web. 26 July 2017.

(16) Vainio H, Kaaks R, and Bianchini F. Weight control and physical activity in cancer prevention: international evaluation of the evidence. Eur J Cancer Prev 2002; 11 Suppl 2: S94-100.

(17) Song M, Giovannucci E. Preventable Incidence and Mortality of Carcinoma Associated With Lifestyle Factors Among White Adults in the United States. JAMA Oncol 2016; 2(9): 1154-61.

(18) Garber JE, Offit K. Hereditary cancer predisposition syndromes. J Clin Oncol 2005; 23(2): 276-92.

(19) Mariotto AB, Yabroff KR, Shao Y, et al. Projections of the cost of cancer care in the United States: 2010-2020. J Natl Cancer Inst 2011; 103(2): 117-28.

(20) "Economic Impact of Cancer." American Cancer Society. N.p., n.d. Web. 02 July 2017.

(21) Reineke K. "10 Statistics On The Cost of Cancer Treatment in America." CancerInsurance.com. N.p., 06 July 2014. Web. 02 July 2017.

(22) Pianin E. "The average out-of-pocket costs for cancer patients can be catastrophic - regardless of health care coverage." Business Insider. Business Insider, 29 Nov. 2016. Web. 02 July 2017.

(23) Andrews A. "Treating with Checkpoint Inhibitors—Figure $1 Million per Patient." American Health & Drug Benefits. Engage Healthcare Communications, LLC, Aug. 2015. Web. 26 July 2017.

CHAPTER 2

What Is Cancer?

"The thief comes to steal, kill, and destroy…"
– John 10:10

Cancer comes from a normal, healthy cell—something good—that is converted into a perversion of that original good thing, something evil. It hides within the body; it tricks and deceives the body, and disrupts all good and natural things within. It is fair to say that cancer is the evil one manifested in a physical form. Cancer comes to steal our health, rob our joy, and destroy our life. This is a spiritual description of a physical process, but the analogy is too fitting to ignore.

I do not believe that God desires for people to get cancer, nor do I think He seals that sentence into anyone's fate. I do not think that cancer is some sort of punishment that God bestows upon the unrighteous, but it can certainly seem that way to cancer sufferers. On the other hand, like many bad things that are the result of living in a fallen world, sometimes a diagnosis of cancer can seem idiopathic, or without an apparent cause or reason.

The goal of medicine is to understand the mechanisms of our fallen world as they relate to our health, and try to rectify them the best we can. For me, that includes addressing the spiritual component to health and well-being, in addition to the medical components. Being mere mortals, however, we often fall short of what the Great Healer is capable of doing. God rewards the faithful, however, and I believe His guidance has revealed a clear path for me and the way I treat cancer patients.

In contrast to Satan, God says that He comes that we may have life and have it to the fullest. I believe that promise, and while I believe that things will never be perfect until we get to heaven, I believe God has provided all we need here on earth to fulfill that promise. Discovering the knowledge necessary to achieve life to the fullest within His creation is my goal as a physician.

What Cancer Is, and How It Develops

Cancer is a very broad term used to describe over 100 different variations of a single disease. While it is a disease of extreme complexity, we can describe it very simply as cells going rogue.

Cells are the basic building blocks for living organisms. It is estimated that the body has between 40 and 100 trillion cells. Each of these cells perform specialized functions in the body, but all contain the same basic structures and mechanisms, such as a surrounding membrane, a nucleus containing DNA, and mitochondria, which produce energy for the cell. Groups of specialized cells form tissues and organs, which perform specific and essential tasks within the body. So while, for example, a cell from the lung performs different functions than a cell from the liver, the individual cells, themselves, share similar characteristics.

One of the similarities that all cells share is their life cycle. This life cycle is divided into three phases: interphase, mitosis, and cytokinesis. Interphase accounts for the majority of a cell's life, as it performs specific, specialized functions and takes in nutrients, preparing to ultimately divide into two daughter cells. Mitosis is the process by which cells begin their duplication, replicating their DNA. Following mitosis, cells enter into cytokinesis, during which time individual cells will split completely into two separate cells, each containing identical copies of the original DNA.

DNA, or deoxyribonucleic acid, is the hereditary information inherent in cells and forms what are called chromosomes. Contained inside the body's 46 chromosomes are instructions for creating and maintaining life. As we know, 23 chromosomes are contributed by Mom and 23 chromosomes are contributed by Dad. These chromosomes are contained inside the nucleus of virtually every cell in the body.

You can think of DNA as the master code for your body. DNA is comprised of chains of four nucleotides, called adenine, cytosine, thymine and guanine. The way these four nucleotides are arranged on the DNA strand is how the information inherent in DNA is coded. The sequence of these four nucleotides along the strands of DNA are read by our body, similar to the way a computer reads binary code consisting of ones and zeros.

Sections of consecutive nucleotides on DNA strands are called genes. If nucleotides are similar to the ones and zeros in binary codes, genes are akin to individual, spelled-out commands. Genes control your physical features, such as height, eye color, and hair color. Genes also control the basic functions of cells, such as energy production within the cell, protein synthesis, and other functions. The collections of genes make up individual chromosomes, which can be thought of as entire computer programs, with many commands and functions.

Our cells are very adept at replicating DNA during the process of mitosis, even though this process of DNA replication occurs many, many times. For the most part, this process is extremely accurate. However, sometimes mistakes occur. Usually, mistakes are corrected when they happen via inherent proofreading mechanisms, but sometimes these errors go undetected.

When genes become altered or damaged, it is known as a mutation. These mutations in the genetic code can affect the subsequent cellular function, and because cellular mitosis creates (mostly) perfect replicas of DNA, those mutations ultimately get passed on to the cellular offspring—referred to as daughter cells. Often times, genetic mutations go unnoticed and affect parts of the genetic code that do not control any sort of vital function. However, because genes control everything a cell does—including its division and lifecycle—if enough mutations occur in the right place, cancer can form.

The Hallmarks of Cancer

Once cancer has begun, we see specific changes in cancer cells that distinguish them from normal, healthy cells. In a landmark study published in the journal *Cell* in 2000, researchers Douglas Hanahan and Robert Weinberg defined the underlying principles common to all cancer cells. There are six principles in total, which distinguish malignant cells from normal cells.

First, cancer cells have self-sufficient growth signals. Normal cells are reliant upon external signals to grow. In contrast, cancer cells stimulate themselves to grow and multiply. Second, cancer cells are insensitive to anti-growth signals. Normal cells have what are known as tumor suppressor genes, which restrict their growth. Cancer cells have altered tumor suppressor genes, which means that the "stop growing" signal is not active.

Third, cancer cells possess the ability to evade apoptosis. Normal cells undergo apoptosis, or programmed cell death, to protect the body. Cancer cells do not undergo this cell suicide, making them immortal. This is related to the fourth characteristic of cancer cells; cancerous cells have limitless replicative potential. Normal cells have a predetermined number of times they can undergo cell division before dying. This is known as the Hayflick limit. Cancer cells do not have this barrier, meaning that they can divide indefinitely (and thus continue to multiply).

The fifth hallmark of cancer cells is that they possess what is known as sustained angiogenesis. Normal cells are restricted by their nearby blood supply. In contrast, cancer cells have the ability to promote angiogenesis, which is the formation of new blood vessels. Cancer cells use this additional blood supply for nourishment to grow and spread. Finally, the sixth hallmark of cancer cells is that they invade nearby tissue and can spread to distant sites, a process known as metastasis. (1)

Why Can Our Body Not Defend Itself Against Cancer?

Our immune system is particularly adept at fighting off infections, including viruses and bacteria. The immune system recognizes these as foreign to the body and creates antibodies that kill these organisms, subsequently protecting us from infection, or fighting infections when they do occur. Many people incorrectly assume that the body's natural defense mechanisms work much the same way in fighting cancer.

This misconception has led to many saying that a strong immune system is the best defense against cancer; the stronger the immune system is, the more likely it is to recognize cancer when it forms and eliminate it accordingly. The thought that our immune system regularly protects us from cancer by eliminating malignant cells before they grow into something life-threatening is an interesting one, but this approach fails to recognize how complex cancer is. The reality is that developing cancer has nothing to do with how strong or weak our immune systems are.

It helps to know a little bit about how the immune system works. Bone marrow, the spongy tissue found deep inside our bones, produces a variety of cells, including white blood cells. These young white blood cells make their way into the lymphatic system. The lymphatic system acts as a training ground for white blood cells and other immune cells. It is here that these cells learn what is foreign, or in other words, what to attack if encountered. They also learn what is self, or what not to attack. Without this distinction, our immune cells would attack normal, healthy tissues, interfering with our body's function. When this process goes awry, we have autoimmune disease in the body.

A lot of specificity goes into training our immune system's cells. For example, some are trained to fight bacteria, some are trained to fight viruses, some are trained to fight fungus, some are trained to fight parasites, and some are trained to fight allergens. The way these cells are trained is that they are exposed to antigens in the lymphatic system. Antigens are structures which are visible on the surface of certain pathogens. When our trained immune cells recognize these antigens within the body, they realize that they are supposed to attack that pathogen, and the body rallies to do that.

Cancer cells, however, are largely devoid of foreign antigens. There is nothing protruding from a cancer cell that signifies to the immune system that it is bad. Cancer, after all, is technically self, and with only very few exceptions, the immune system recognizes no distinction between a cancer cell and a normal cell.

Once cancer has begun, there really is no way to reverse the process; cancer simply must be killed. Ultimately, our immune system is ill-equipped to fight cancer the way it fights infections or other diseases. The answer to preventing and treating cancer does not rely on having a stronger immune system, although that is an important component to overall health. A healthy immune system simply does not mean you can prevent cancer from forming, and strengthening your immune system following a cancer diagnosis will not cure the disease.

Viewing Cancer as a Genetic Disease

The last few decades of research have centered largely on the genetic component of cancer. Since it is understood that a mutation in the genetic material triggers the formation of cancer, most of the research into cancer has centered on understanding the mechanisms that are the result of damaged DNA. In the last 20 years, researchers have made tremendous strides in understanding the genetics of cancer.

This focus, however, is somewhat shortsighted because it does little to address what still lies at the root of the problem. While we understand that genetic mutations are an important part of how cancer develops, and are responsible for giving cancer cells their aggressive behavior, little has been done to address what *causes* those genetic mutations to begin with.

This might be a big reason why cancer prevention is rarely the emphasis when it comes to our discussion on cancer. Instead, what is communicated is that the genetic mutations that lead to cancer happen largely without any reason, and are thus outside our ability to influence or change.

Genes and Your Risk for Cancer

Another problem with exclusively viewing cancer as a genetic disease is that by and large, the public thinks that if cancer is "in their family," there is a strong likelihood they will develop it, too. Conversely, many falsely assume that because they have no familial history of cancer, they are not at risk. Both assumptions, however, do not stack up with what we see as far as the incidence of cancer.

The best data suggests that 6-8% of all cancers are genetic in origin. It is true that we have seen certain inherited genes that have a correlation to the development of certain cancers, such as the BRCA1 and BRCA2 genes in cases of breast and ovarian cancers. However, the presence of these genes does not guarantee one will develop cancer. Regardless, many who learn that they have inherited these genes live in fear of developing cancer, to the point that many women undergo radical mastectomies and hysterectomies upon learning they have these specific genes.

Ultimately, the small subset of inherited genetic triggers does not account for the other 92% of cancers we see. All of the genetic knowledge we have gained, and all the strides we have made in understanding those mechanisms simply tell an incomplete story. The focus on the genetic component of cancer has, instead, detracted from what causes genetic mutations in the first place.

Furthermore, it is important to realize that genetic mutations that are passed through families and increase the risk of cancer are still likely the result of some previous insult to genetic material. These genetic abnormalities, themselves, do not necessarily constitute the *cause* of the disease. In other words, the breast cancer a woman experiences possibly started with a mutation incurred by her grandmother that was subsequently passed down. What caused the disease was not actually the genetic mutation itself, but whatever instigated it; the change in genetic material was simply the first domino knocked over, so to speak. This is an important distinction, because it speaks to what I feel is a significant flaw in the way we view cancer.

The Toxic Bucket

One of the biggest problems with cancer has always been that because it is such a complex disease, any new evidence discovered that sheds light on its development, progression, or treatment immediately co-opts all the attention of everyone within the scientific community. First, it was radiation therapy in the beginning of the 20th century. Forty years later, it was chemotherapy, and twenty five years after that, it was the study of genetics. We have collectively put a lot of research in money into these areas, and not without some success.

We have progressed exponentially in the field of radiology. Chemotherapy is more effective than ever before, and we have learned how to mitigate some of its terrible side effects. Today, we know so much about the genetic mechanisms that drive cancer development. However, there is comparatively little research into—and little discussion about—what causes those genetic mutations to begin with.

This is a problem, because what we are missing may have more to do with what causes cancer to begin with than genetics, alone. If our best guess is that 8% of cancers are genetic in origin, we can safely assume that perhaps there must be some sort of environmental factors at play in the other 92% of cancers. We have focused so strongly on understanding the genetic mechanism of cancer development that we miss what set that mechanism into motion.

Normal, healthy cells all endure a certain level of bombardment over the course of their lives. At a certain point however, they can become overwhelmed by the repeated damage they incur from their environment. It is helpful to think of this as a bucket; if the bucket continues to get filled, eventually, it is going to overflow.

Each individual has a different sized bucket, so to speak, and can sustain a different amount of toxic bombardment. This is why some people might get lung cancer, and others can smoke well into their old age and die of "natural causes." For everyone, however, there likely exists a threshold; at some point our cells cannot sustain the repeated damaged incurred from their environment. The environment our cells are continuously bathed in eventually takes its toll on the genetic material inside our cells if that environment is less than optimal.

There are a variety of ways we can create toxic environments for our cells. One of the primary ways we do this is through exposure to carcinogenic agents. Many people are aware that cigarettes, asbestos, and ionizing radiation can cause cancer. But the list of known carcinogens extends far beyond what many people would initially assume.

The International Agency for Research on Cancer (IARC) is part of the World Health Organization (WHO), and is one of the groups tasked with identifying causes of cancer. Among its many goals, the IARC seeks to identify possible carcinogens. They have developed the most notable, scaled classification systems for identifying carcinogens.

The classification is broken down into four groups: Group 1 is definitely carcinogenic to humans; group 2A is probably carcinogenic to humans; group 2B is possibly carcinogenic to humans; group 3 is unclassifiable as to carcinogenicity in humans; and group 4 is probably not carcinogenic to humans. Other groups, such as the National Toxicology Program (NTP) and the Environmental Protection Agency (EPA), have similar classification systems denoting carcinogenicity of certain products, chemicals, compounds, medicines, and infectious agents.

The IARC has tested over 900 agents; of those, 112 are listed in group 1, or carcinogenic to humans. Another 75 are listed in group 2A, or probably carcinogenic to humans. Certainly, the knowledge of these is a good start. What is concerning, however, is that many of the agents listed by the IARC in groups 1 and 2 are fairly common contaminants of our environment.

A good example is the pesticide, glyphosate. Glyphosate is one of the most commonly used herbicides in the world, and has been used since the 1970s. Glyphosate is so widely used, because many crops (including many staple crops, such as corn and soy) have been genetically engineered to be resistant to its use, meaning glyphosate can be doused on these crops without fear of harming the crops themselves, only the unwanted weeds. Glyphosate is absorbed into the plants it is used on, meaning it is impossible to rinse or scrub off.

Repeatedly, we were told that glyphosate was safe, but in 2015, the World Health Organization placed glyphosate in group 2A, designating it as probably carcinogenic to humans. Those at highest risk are typically those who handle the herbicide regularly, such as farm workers. While we are told there is little risk for those of us who are simply exposed to glyphosate via our diet, we do not have long-term studies to substantiate this. Glyphosate is a good example of how chemicals that are well documented as carcinogenic are still prevalent in our environment.

Without speculating too much, the toxic bucket analogy still likely applies in the case of chemicals like glyphosate. A small drip over a long time can fill up a bucket. A lifetime's worth of exposure to glyphosate, coupled with the hundreds of other known carcinogens that regularly contaminate our environment, is bound to eventually take a toll on our cells. Thus, it is not surprising that cancer risk increases with age.

Chemical Bloom

The word, *chemical,* has a dirty connotation to it, although it is not a bad word in and of itself. Everything you see, smell, taste, or touch consists of a chemical composition, from the healthiest vegetable, to the water you drink, to the computer you use. Even your own body has its unique chemistry. We are surrounded by chemicals.

Until recently, however, our bodies were not inundated with the volume of chemicals that we see today. The war effort in both World War I and World War II led to the discovery and use of many new chemical compounds. Following World War II, we saw rapid increases in technology and consumer products which were largely a result of research and development from the war effort. Since then, there has been an exponential increase in the number of consumer products brought to market, and subsequently, an enormous amount of new chemicals released into our environment. It is estimated that since that time, there have been more that 84,000 unique chemicals brought to market or introduced into the environment. As little as 1% have been fully tested for safety. This is a staggering statistic, with potentially severe ramifications to our health. (2)

The issue has become the enormous volume of unnatural chemicals that we come into contact with every day. Many—if not most—of these are likely harmless. The issue really becomes that we do not fully understand what the long-term effects are of our chemically-laden environment. In spite of the hundreds of chemicals the IARC and other agencies have deemed carcinogenic or probably carcinogenic, there remains a tremendous volume of chemicals available in some form on the market today that are either untested, or not fully tested, for carcinogenicity. Moreover, the issue is not simply whether a chemical is inherently carcinogenic, but also the dose which is required to cause damage to our cells. We simply do not know what the long-term effects of these kinds of exposure are.

Simply thinking about what we come in contact with today versus 100 years ago—from the building materials in our homes, to the cleaning chemicals used in our homes and workspaces, to the industrial chemicals necessary for our phones, automobiles and computers and other modern conveniences, to the cosmetics we use—we are bombarded with chemical exposures we would have never experienced 100 years ago. Today, even our foods contain ingredients we cannot even pronounce. In comparison to what our ancestors experienced, the volume of chemical exposure we experience is staggering.

It is impossible for us to have an understanding of what the long term consequences are for these exposures, especially when we do not have a full understanding of the effects these chemicals can have on our body. It does not take a statistician to realize that as the volume of available chemicals has increased, so have cancer rates. Is there a correlation between the two? It is not definitive, but it certainly seems probable.

It is important to note that research lags far behind bringing many products to market, and any sort of regulatory change lags even farther behind that. We have all seen the advertisements from the 1950s, with doctors in white coats smoking cigarettes, recommending this brand or the other, and touting the health benefits of smoking. Everyone from soldiers, to businessmen, to even pregnant women smoked! Merely a few decades later, we realized how dangerous cigarettes actually were and that they caused multiple kinds of cancers.

Many will recall, however, the cigarette companies fought tooth and nail to prevent that knowledge from being discovered. Many cigarette companies funded their own "research" into the harmful effects of cigarettes. Many of these studies were deemed inconclusive, or stated that cigarettes were not addictive and do not cause harm. It was only after years of litigation that cigarette companies were legally compelled to admit wrongdoing, pay damages, and issue warnings on their products.

We know invariably that cigarettes are addictive and cause cancer, among other health problems. The tobacco companies knew this too. In spite of the fact they knew their product was causing tremendous harm, they chose to act in the best interest of their company. If this was the case years ago for big tobacco, one may assume it remains the case for large corporations today; they certainly are not going to implicate their own products in causing cancer, nor will they likely voluntarily conduct long-term research into the health effects of their wares, particularly if large sums of money are to be made in the meantime.

On the other hand, the response from the conventional medical community about this issue of overwhelming chemical exposure is tepid, at best. The reason conventional medicine does not recognize—or at least, does not vocalize—the huge concern associated with the volume of chemical exposure people are subjected to is because it has not necessarily been *proven* that any of these chemicals are harmful. In other words, we have not tested a certain chemical for safety, so we do not know whether it is safe, therefore we cannot tell you that it is unsafe.

It is time to use more common sense when it comes to what we expose ourselves to, particularly as that exposure relates to cancer. It is simply imprudent to wait around for decades for scientists to conclude that a specific chemical is dangerous and causes cancer.

Toxic Stress, Toxic Lifestyle

We have all been told that mitigating stress in our life is important. There is evidence that high stress lifestyles can induce a variety of health problems, including cancer.

No one likely took this theory to its logical extreme more than Dr. Ryke Hamer. Dr. Hamer was a German doctor who developed a theory on the origins of cancer. Born in 1935, Dr. Hamer received his medical license at 26 and spent the next few years working in the university clinics of Tubingen and Heidleberg. In 1972, Dr. Hamer completed his specialization in internal medicine at the age of 37.

Dr. Hamer's son was accidentally shot in 1978; four months later, he died from complications related to the gunshot wound. Understandably,

Dr. Hamer and his family were devastated. Shortly thereafter, Dr. Hamer developed testicular cancer. Suspecting there was some link between his cancer and the emotional trauma related to his son's sudden, unexpected death, Dr. Hamer began research into the connection between life trauma and the development of disease, particularly cancer.

What he purported to find was that traumatic life events set biochemical changes in motion that could lead to the development of cancer and other diseases. He developed this theory to the extent that he believed he could predict exactly what kind of cancer, and where in the body it would develop if he knew what particular life trauma had occurred in a patient's life.

Dr. Hamer would call this area of research German New Medicine. His theories are very controversial, so much so that his license was revoked by the German authorities. Many of the components of German New Medicine are unproven and untested. Regardless, there are many who still believe Dr. Hamer's theories to be accurate. Regardless of how controversial Dr. Hamer and German New Medicine is, his work certainly underscores some of what our own science has said about the causes of cancer.

The body's natural stress mechanisms have a natural, specific role that they play, such as the secretion of certain hormones, like cortisol. The problem lies within the fact that our biochemistry has done a poor job at keeping up with our modern lifestyle. Before the advent of modern life, stress hormones were triggered only as necessary, often during "fight or flight" situations. These bodily processes and functions were highly beneficial for our ancestors, who would find themselves in life or death situations far more than we do. For example, if you were fleeing a predator, or facing said predator in a fight, the heightened awareness and boost of adrenaline were very beneficial for your chance at survival.

The problem has becomes that because of our fast-paced, overstressed lifestyles, we constantly bathe our cells in a cocktail of stress hormones. These stress hormones, however, can become a toxic agent in our bodies when maintained at heightened levels over long periods of time. We know that this can have an effect on our genes, much the way exposure to toxic, foreign chemical agents can. If we couple this with the emotional trauma everyone experiences as a part of the course of life, it can be argued that the pressures we inflict on our own body via stress can damage our own DNA, leading to cancer.

Regardless, the mitigation of stress is seldom talked about in the discussion on what causes cancer and how we can prevent it.

Natural Exposures

Cancer is not exclusively the result of man-made influences, although it can be argued that manmade influences play a very significant role. We know, however, that there are natural forces and agents that have a proven ability to cause cancer. Among these are ultraviolet light from the sun, certain toxins made by fungi such as aflatoxins, and certain infectious agents like *Helicobacter pylori* or human papilloma virus (HPV).

The fact that natural carcinogens exist serves to underscore two main points. First, it provides proof that cancer is not exclusively a relatively new, man-made disease, something many people wrongfully espouse. Cancer has existed for millennia, something autopsies of ancient Egyptian mummies revealed. Operating under the assumption that genetic insults that lead to cancer are largely the result of external or environmental factors, we know our ancestors would have been exposed to many of these agents, such as UV light, viruses, mycotoxins, and other infective agents. Combined with genetic predisposition, life stressors, and other factors, it only makes sense that cancer is not exclusively a manmade disease and has existed long before our ability to diagnose it.

Second, many people in the holistic medicine community typically want to point the finger exclusively at man-made causes of cancer and demonize anything manmade that can treat cancer. There are plenty of so-called natural compounds that are just as dangerous—and carcinogenic—as man-made agents. This is extremely shortsighted thinking; while conventional oncology certainly has its flaws, and natural medicine certainly has its benefits that often go unrecognized by mainstream scientists, it is time to find some middle ground.

Regardless, in light of the cancer trends we have seen over the past century, it is fair to point the finger at a variety of man-made agents as the overwhelming cause of cancer.

Malignancy in Order to Survive

Let's return to the cell. All of our cells are surrounded by a cell membrane made of cholesterol and fat. That membrane performs a variety of tasks, including giving a cell its structure. It also acts as the gatekeeper for the cell; the cell membrane decides what comes in and out of the cell.

The result of all the stressors we have talked about—including man-made agents, natural agents, and emotional stressors—is that the cell membrane becomes inflamed. We can measure this level of inflammation with a blood test called the C-reactive protein test, or CRP. The CRP level provides us a marker for cellular inflammation. What we see over time is that levels of CRP tend to rise, and our cells become more and more inflamed.

We know that as our cells become more inflamed, they do not function as well, and they become progressively weaker. They do not create ATP (the energy currency of the cell) and they fail to perform their function optimally. Whether it is a cell helping your heart to beat, or a cell that gives your skin its structure, or a cell that functions for metabolism, the inflamed cell ceases to function as it should. It takes progressively more energy and effort for the cell to perform its function until, ultimately, the cell reaches its capacity. This should ideally trigger apoptosis, whereby this damaged cell kills itself, in order to protect the overall functioning of the body.

Other times, however, the cell can alter its genes in order to stay alive indefinitely. The altering of genes becomes a survival mechanism for the cell to withstand the bombardment it continually receives. Here, we see the cell losing its predetermined lifespan. This is where we see the crossover from a normal cell to a cancerous cell. It is at this point when the cell's genetic material is altered.

In the same way that our toxic bucket can only hold so much before overflowing, our cells can only withstand so much bombardment in the form of natural, man-made, and emotional stressors before something must change within the cell itself—apoptosis or mutation. For everyone, that threshold is different, but ultimately, everyone is at risk for reaching their limit, and thus, seeing a transformation from healthy cell into cancerous cell.

Cancer as a Metabolic Disease

Conventional oncologists and cancer researchers have placed the focus on the genetic component to cancer, and this has been the paradigm for years. In their view, cancer is a genetic disease, and this view predominantly informs their approach to treating cancer as well as the research that goes into cancer.

Integrative oncology maintains a different view of the nature of what cancer fundamentally is. We have described how outside influences, including natural and man-made agents, are often the cause of the genetic insults that instigate the formation of cancer. In addition, we have described the role that prolonged stress may play in the process of cancer development. All things accounted for, we know that genetics can only be blamed for less than 10% of all cancers. Even then, genetic cancers are likely the result of genetic damage initially incurred by environmental factors, and then passed down from parents to children.

I approach cancer from a different perspective. Cancer is much less of a genetic disease than it is a metabolic disease; the genetic component to cancer is merely a result of our cells' metabolic processes—the processes by which our cells make energy—becoming interfered with, or compromised, by a variety of factors and agents. This view, however, is not without precedent, and has been supported by a variety of researchers through the years.

Among those is Dr. Otto Warburg (1883-1970). Dr. Warburg was a German physiologist and medical doctor. In 1931, he received the Nobel Prize in Physiology or Medicine, a prize for which he was nominated for 46 times. Dr. Warburg did quite a bit to advance our understanding of cancer. What ultimately earned him the Nobel Prize was discovering the way cancer cells make energy, or ATP.

Dr. Warburg wrote that, "The first phase (of cancer cells' origination) is the irreversible damage to respiration (metabolism)." (3) Normal, healthy cells are very good at producing ATP. Our healthy cells go through a multi-step process to create energy, and typically produce around 32-36 units of ATP. Cancer cannot do that; it is not nearly as efficient. Cancer goes through a very small part of that metabolic process—only the first step, known as glycolysis. During glycolysis, a cancer cell essentially burns sugar for energy, and it only produces 2 units of ATP. This is the primary way by which cancer can make energy, and it is a very labor-intensive process. It is also a very important distinction between a normal, healthy cell, and a cancer cell.

This discovery led to some of the ways we can find cancer in the body; on a PET scan, we observe cancer cells consuming radioactive glucose at a rate far faster than healthy cells. This also has implications on how integrative oncology can successfully treat cancer, which is covered in the next chapters.

Dr. Warburg was convinced that the damage to cellular metabolism was at the root of cancer development. He wrote that, "If the explanation of a vital process is its reduction to physics and chemistry, there is today no other explanation for the origin of cancer cells, either special or general. From this point of view, mutation and carcinogenic agent are not alternatives, but empty words, unless metabolically specified." In other words, what Dr. Warburg believed his research pointed to was that genetic mutations were the result of a cell's metabolism being compromised.

This is essentially what we see when cells ultimately reach their threshold of inflammation and mutate in order to survive; once a cell becomes overburdened in a toxic environment, whether the factors that lead to that inflammation threshold are natural agents, man-made agents, or stress-induced agents, its energy production is compromised, and the cell mutates in order to survive.

Dr. Warburg made other important discoveries related to cancer. Along with his discovery that cancer cells preferentially consume glucose for energy, Dr. Warburg also realized that cancer cells do not thrive in oxygen-rich environments. Hypoxia, or lack of oxygen, does much to contribute to the creation of cancer cells. Another important metabolic feature of cancer, he discovered, is that cancer's energy production results in a significant amount of lactic acid. This is why we see a lot of acidity in and around cancer cells, and one reason why many talk about the importance of pH, or alkalinity vs. acidity when it comes to cancer.

Building on Warburg

For many years, much of Dr. Warburg's work was cast aside, despite the fact that it was fundamental to our development of understanding of cancer. Much of the interest in treating cancer was diverted to chemotherapy in the 1940s, and then genetics in the latter half of the 20th century. In recent years, however, there has been somewhat of a revived academic interest in Dr. Warburg's work.

Dr. Thomas Seyfried of Boston College is one of the researchers who have built upon the work of Dr. Warburg. His research has led him to agree with Dr. Warburg, in that cancer can largely be viewed as a metabolic disease. In a study published in 2009, Dr. Seyfried concluded that, "All of the major hallmarks of the disease (cancer) can be linked to impaired mitochondrial function...the abundance of somatic genomic abnormalities found in the majority of cancers can arise as a secondary consequence of mitochondrial dysfunction. Once established somatic genomic instability can contribute to further mitochondrial defects and to the metabolic inflexibility of the cancer cell." (4)

Dr. Seyfried believes that many of the hallmarks of cancer, such as the genetic abnormalities, are all downstream of the primary issue, which is the interference of cellular metabolism, primarily through the repeated damage to mitochondria, where cells produce energy.

In light of the fact that genetics play a less pronounced role than we have been led to believe, and that we know a variety of agents can elevate levels of inflammation in cellular habitats, and that inflammation ultimately leads to the degradation of the cell and its ability to produce energy, the view that cancer is more metabolic than genetic comes into sharper focus. Our toxic bucket may overflow when our cells' energy production is disrupted, causing our cells to mutate simply in order to survive. The research of Dr. Warburg, Dr. Seyfried, and others certainly seems to point in this direction. The continued expansion of this work is important, because it opens the door to many methods that can potentially assist us in both successfully treating cancer, and ideally preventing it in the first place.

Genetics vs. Epigenetics

Many people believe that they are somehow bound to their genes, and that subsequently they have very little control over their bodies or their health. This is an idea that has largely been perpetuated by conventional science and medicine, but not always for the better. Many people believe that if they "have cancer in their families," there is nothing they can do to prevent it; many wind up living in fear of getting a diagnosis, often for their entire lives.

Many people who have genetic predispositions to cancer, though, never get cancer. The mechanisms behind this are not fully understood; there is simply too much we still do not know to understand why this is. However, feeling as if your health is exclusively bound to your genetics is simply misguided. The fact is that you do have significant control over many aspects of your health. Certainly, there are aspects of your genetics that you cannot change; you cannot biologically increase your height, change your hair or eye color, or your fingerprint. What we do know, however, is that our environment can have a profound impact on our genetics. There is a mounting body of scientific evidence to support this.

The field of epigenetics—a term that literally means, in *addition* to changes in genetic sequence—has become one of the most intriguing areas of research in genetics. The premise of epigenetics is that the expression of certain genes is contingent upon a host of external factors. Bob Weinhold writes, "Today, a wide variety of illnesses, behaviors and other health indicators already have some level of evidence linking them with epigenetic mechanisms, including cancers of all types..." (5)

A study on the relationship between cancer and genetics published in 2012 stated that, "Cancer initiation and progression is controlled by both genetic and epigenetic events. The complexity of carcinogenesis cannot be accounted for by genetic alterations alone but also involves epigenetic changes." (6) Genes can be thought of as a light switch, which can either be turned on or off. Our genes are constantly changing and adapting to their environment, even on an hour by hour basis. Our cells, and subsequently our genes, can be subjected to a hospitable environment, with good conditions, or an inhospitable environment, with less than optimal conditions. By creating beneficial conditions in the body, it is possible to essentially "turn off" bad genes, and "turn on" good genes. These conditions are highly influenced by our choices via nutrition, stress, how much we exercise, and many other factors.

This means that it is no longer acceptable to think that we are beholden so strongly to our genetics. In a study published in 2010, Sikhar Sharma writes, "Global changes in the epigenetic landscape are a hallmark of cancer. The initiation and progression of cancer, traditionally seen as a genetic disease, is now realized to involve epigenetic abnormalities along with genetic alterations." (7)

Much of the research is arriving at a similar consensus; there are factors outside of DNA itself that dictate how our genes are expressed. This is in stark contrast to the attitude held by many researchers, doctors, and particularly oncologists, for many, many years—many of whom still hold onto this antiquated belief today. The implications of our study of epigenetics are profound. The question then becomes, what is it, specifically, that we must do in order to create a beneficial environment for our genes?

The field of epigenetics is still a very new area of research, but the evidence now points toward the fact that we have far more control over our genes than we once thought. This revelation is exciting and empowering; further research into epigenetics is needed, but the preliminary data this field of study has produced shows we are moving in the right direction.

(1) Hanahan D, Weinberg RA. The Hallmarks of Cancer. Cell 2000; 100 (1): 57-70.

(2) Urbina, Ian. "Think Those Chemicals Have Been Tested?" The New York Times. The New York Times, 13 Apr 2013. Web. 26 July 2017.

(3) Warburg OH. On The Origin of Cancer Cells" Science 1956; 123(3191): 309-14.

(4) Seyfried TN, Shelton LM. Cancer as a Metabolic Disease. Nutr Metab (Lond) 2010; 7: 7.

(5) Weinhold B. Epigenetics: the science of change. Environ Health Perspect 2006; 114(3): A160-7.

(6) Sharma S, Kelly TK, Jones PA. Epigenetics in cancer. Carcinogenesis 2010; 31(1): 27-36.

(7) Kanwal R, Gupta S. Epigenetic modifications in cancer. Clin Genet 2012; 81(4): 303-11.

CHAPTER 3

What Is Integrative Oncology?

"Good, better, best. Never let it rest.
'Til your good is better and your better is best."
— St. Jerome

Integrative oncology combines the best aspects of two seemingly contradictory branches of medicine: conventional medicine, also referred to as allopathic, Western, or modern medicine; and alternative medicine, also referred to as natural or holistic medicine. With regard to cancer, an integrative approach gives us a wider palette of therapies and treatments. It is a necessary step forward in the progression of how we treat a disease which does not respond well to purely conventional or alternative approaches alone.

These shortcomings are evidenced by three important facts, which we discussed previously: First, cancer is quickly becoming the number one killer of people in developed countries, overtaking heart disease. Second, the lifetime risk for any person developing cancer has increased dramatically; today, the risk is nearly 1 out of 2. Finally, despite billions of dollars spent to find a cure, the death rate from cancer has not significantly improved.

Something must be done to address this. Undoubtedly, addressing the issue of cancer in its entirety—from how we view the disease, to our discussion on prevention, to how we treat it—requires looking outside of what conventional oncology has to offer. We have come a long way, but we still have a long way to go.

Problems with the Current Standard of Care

As it stands today, we know more about cancer than ever before in history. We have made tremendous strides in the field of radiology, in the development of new chemotherapy and immunotherapy drugs, and in the precision with which we perform surgical procedures. The standards of care today are evidenced-based with an overwhelming amount of good science and rigorous studies to back up their use.

However, this does not mean that the way that we treat cancer is not without its shortcomings. Particularly, in light of the disappointing statistics covered in chapter 1, we realize that for all of our research and knowledge, we still are not winning the war on cancer. In fact, we are losing badly. As it turns out, there is still plenty we do not know, and we stand to learn a lot. While conventional oncology today does all it can within its purview, there is more that can be done. It is my sincere belief, based on my training and clinical practice, that we can do far better.

To start with, it is helpful to know what the process looks like for someone who is diagnosed with cancer. For those of you who have already undergone cancer treatment, this process will likely be very familiar to you.

If you are a woman, and you feel a lump in your breast, you will hopefully have either your OB-GYN, family doctor, or internist examine the lump. Your doctor will likely order a mammogram and ultrasound, and if it still looks suspicious, you will typically have a biopsy to confirm cancer. If the biopsy is positive, your doctor will refer you to a medical oncologist and a surgical oncologist. You might also be referred to a radiation oncologist. The order of referral might vary in some degree.

Sometimes, the medical oncologist will coordinate both surgery and radiation consults.

Often, the process between diagnosis and treatment moves very quickly. Following their first trip to a medical oncologist, many patients are scheduled to begin treatment within a few days. This haste is largely because the protocols for cancer treatment are well established within conventional oncology. For example, if you have a certain type of breast cancer, and it is at a specific stage, there is what is known as first-line treatment. This will include treatments that are known to work best for this specific kind of cancer at this stage. If that series of treatments is unsuccessful, your oncologist will likely recommend second-line treatments, which entails a different combination also thought to have efficacy against your particular cancer.

This can be thought of as "flow chart" medicine, or "cookbook" medicine. It is very much a one-size-fits-all approach to treating cancer. There is a general lack of personalization or tailoring of treatment to each patient. This may be an efficient way of treating cancer if your intent is to treat as many patients as possible, but it certainly generalizes the entire patient population and makes assumptions about commonalities between patients. While studies are important methods for predicting treatment responses for entire populations, they are not necessarily applicable to each individual patient. After all, we now know through genetic analysis of cancerous tissues and cells that each cancer case is as unique as a fingerprint.

As a result of this individuality, each case comes with its own share of hurdles and challenges. No two cancer cases are exactly alike, just as no two patients are exactly alike. By denying this, conventional oncology probably affects many of its outcomes negatively. This is not to say that conventional oncology does not receive good outcomes, necessarily. However, we have learned that by tailoring treatment to the individual patient, you are able to target cancer in a way that most effectively treats it, minimize collateral damage, and give the best chance at a good outcome. With that said, there is no such thing as a sure thing in treating cancer. Our goal, regardless of the type and stage of cancer, should be to improve the chances of success as much as possible!

What You Will and Will Not Hear From Your Oncologist

In the short period of time between diagnosis and the start of treatment, there are a couple of things that you will hear from your oncologist. He or she will likely discuss prognosis and chances of success based on existing data. Surgery will likely be discussed, if you are thought to be a good candidate. He or she will discuss the best course of chemotherapy, what side effects to be prepared for, and how to best mitigate them. Often, your oncologist will go ahead and write prescriptions for drugs that help with the side effects of chemotherapy and/or immunotherapy, such as nausea, vomiting, diarrhea, and fatigue. Finally, if radiation is appropriate, that will be discussed as well. You will get referrals and a schedule for upcoming treatments within this standard of care.

What you will most certainly not hear about is anything related to nutrition, supplementation, exercise, stress reduction, or any other natural or alternative therapies. At the most, your oncologist might ask you about the supplements you are taking, if any, for fear of them interfering with the chemotherapy treatment or other prescription drugs.

There is some confusion when it comes to many oncologists' knowledge of supplements and how they work. Vitamin C provides some good examples of the limitations of many oncologists' knowledge in regard to supplements. For a long time, it was assumed that antioxidants should be avoided by people who were undergoing chemotherapy treatment, because it was thought that antioxidants would counteract the pro-oxidant effect of chemotherapy. This is something that has been debunked; a wide variety of studies confirm that antioxidants do not interfere with treatments like chemotherapy and radiation, and actually protect healthy cells from the side effects of treatment. (1) Yet, many oncologists cling to the idea that patients should never mix antioxidant supplementation with chemotherapy and/or radiation for fear of diminishing their effects on the cancer being treated.

Similarly, many oncologists erroneously believe that high dose vitamin C should not be part of a treatment protocol, because it is an antioxidant. Aside from the fact that antioxidants do not interfere with chemotherapy, vitamin C actually becomes a *pro-oxidant* in the high doses we use in intravenous vitamin C. These examples only underscore the lack of knowledge many oncologists have when it comes to supplements, yet they still tend to authoritatively discourage their use.

As far as diet is concerned, no nutritional information is typically offered by conventional oncology. In fact, if you ask your oncologist about diet, most will tell you that it does not matter what you eat, at least as far as your treatment is concerned. This is inexcusable for any physician who claims to practice evidence-based medicine! At most, you will get warnings about losing too much weight during treatment. Anything in addition to that, in terms of diet, is ignored.

Sometimes, an oncologist will refer patients to a nutritionist. Sadly, much of the advice issued by nutritionists is fairly poor, particularly when it comes to a diet that would potentially help fight against cancer. Most of the information given is very basic. Their recommendations center around antiquated dietary recommendations such as the food guide pyramid with which we are all familiar. None of the advice given necessarily pertains to how to use nutrition to best improve cancer treatment outcomes.

There are a variety of reasons why you get so little by way of nutritional information from an oncology clinic. There is the oft-heard trope that doctors only receive 2 hours of nutritional training in medical school. That is a bit of an exaggeration. In total, doctors receive about 25 lecture hours in medical school regarding nutrition, but it typically overlaps with areas such as biochemistry. Most of what doctors learn fails to go beyond what you would hear from a general nutritionist. When a doctor moves into residency and fellowship, there is virtually no discussion on diet and nutrition; at best, it is minimal. The lack of emphasis on nutrition during medical training is one reason why doctors, and particularly oncologists, do not place a great deal of value on it.

A 2014 survey of physicians in residency training supported this notion. A total of 94% of resident physicians surveyed agreed that it was their obligation to discuss nutrition with their patients, but only 14% felt adequately trained to provide nutritional counseling. (2)

Unfortunately, an attitude shift regarding nutrition seems to occur between residency training in internal medicine, which all oncologists must complete, and fellowship training in oncology. If you ask most oncologists if they feel that nutrition is an important aspect of cancer treatment, they will tell you that it is not. Thus, oncologists tend to de-emphasize nutrition because they lack the expertise in it as well as the appreciation for it. Many believe that there is no scientific basis for nutrition's role in this setting. This belief, however, is not supported by existing evidence. Certainly, many oncologists are aware of the studies that suggest that diet can prevent cancer, but when it comes to treating cancer, the literature clearly shows that nutrition plays a key role. (3, 4)

The likely reason why doctors fail to emphasize nutrition as part of a comprehensive cancer-fighting regimen is because they only look at the large, well-funded studies that show up in the major medical journals or get presented at the major conferences. The amount of funding it takes to conduct and publish a high quality nutrition study is quite significant, and there simply have not been many studies conducted on this scale to provide the conclusive evidence many oncologists look for. The only studies which receive that sort of funding—either from the public or private sector—typically only focus on improving the existing standards of care for medical, surgical, and radiological treatments. Therefore, most oncologists only hear about new chemotherapy or immunotherapy drugs, or advancements in radiology, genetics, or surgical procedures. While these treatments are valuable tools in the arsenal, and research on them is essential, they only represent a portion of the tools we should have in our tool chest.

The fact that we do not have randomized, double-blind, placebo-controlled studies on the efficacy of diet is frustrating, simply because there is some good evidence that diet and nutrition play a key role in cancer treatment. However, it serves to underscore perhaps one of the biggest flaws in conventional oncology: many in the field possess an inability to accept anything that has not been taught to them as the standard of care. Moreover, most will not even entertain the notion that other modalities might be beneficial in some regard—all while watching many of their patients die.

We are still left not knowing what we do not know. I am reminded of one of my program directors, who told me something as a first-year resident physician that I will never forget. He told me that he was not impressed by what I know, but rather, that I know what I do not know. He went on to explain that the most dangerous physicians are the ones who are oblivious to what they do not know, and as a result, they do not see what they are missing. When this occurs, mistakes and omissions occur and patients can have negative outcomes.

It is a scary thought to reflect on what we do not know when it comes to optimal cancer treatment. What we know for a fact—including chemotherapy, radiation, immunotherapy, and surgery, for example— we know very well. We know how they work, and in many cases, how well they are likely to work. But we are clearly missing something, as evidenced by the lack of significant progress in treatment outcomes.

In my presentations, I often describe the typical approach to cancer treatment as looking through a periscope. We can see a lot when we look through a periscope—far more than if we only looked underwater. But the fact remains that we certainly cannot see everything. The danger lies in assuming that what we see through the periscope is all that exists. In reality, there is an entire world out there that we cannot see if we limit our view to the periscope. Although we might not be able to see those additional landscapes as well as we would like, we can still see a lot if we are just willing to look. And my belief is that we will really like what we see!

Integrative Oncology

What integrative oncology seeks to do is pick up where conventional oncology leaves off, and improve upon it greatly by incorporating evidence-based therapies from the natural and alternative realms. The value lies in offering a best-of-both-worlds approach to treating cancer. We do this by utilizing treatments which are within the standard of care, as well as many which are not necessarily within those standards, but have shown some level of promise against cancer. We do not—and must not—abandon evidence-based medicine, but we should be willing to evaluate that evidence through a different lens.

In my postgraduate training, I was fortunate enough to have the opportunity to work closely with Barry Boyd, MD, a medical oncologist and assistant clinical professor at Yale University School of Medicine. In addition to his conventional training in oncology, Dr. Boyd also has a master's degree in nutrition, and is Director of Cancer Nutrition at Yale. Dr. Boyd combines the conventional standard of care treatments with science-based nutrition and supplementation. He was the first oncologist I had met who was genuinely open to interventions outside of the standard of care. In contrast to most oncologists who tell patients that nutrition does not matter, Dr. Boyd actually spent time discussing diet and supplementation with patients. During the time I spent with Dr. Boyd in the hospital and in his clinic, I noticed that his patients seemed to tolerate full-dose chemotherapy and radiation better than other doctors' patients did, and also tended to have better outcomes overall. Dr. Boyd opened my eyes to the powerful role that nutrition and supplementation can have in a cancer treatment plan. My experience learning from Dr. Boyd created a thirst for integrative cancer treatments that I have not been able to quench in the years since.

Similarities between Conventional and Integrative Oncology

In the interest of taking a best-of-both-worlds approach, integrative oncology incorporates many of the same diagnostic and treatment tools as does conventional oncology. Diagnostically, we really do not change anything. Patients still need to have appropriate biopsies. We embrace biopsies and conventional lab testing such as tumor markers (for example, CA 15-3, CA 19-9, CA 27.29, CA 125, CEA, AFP, etc.). Appropriate imaging, such as PET scans, CT scans, MRIs, and X-rays, is important as well. Getting a proper diagnosis of cancer is a critical first step in treating cancer, and having all of the pertinent information using as many tools as possible is critical to knowing what we are dealing with. It makes no sense going into battle without specific information as to who our foe is.

Once a proper diagnosis of cancer is made, including its stage, we begin to discuss treatment options. In my integrative oncology practice, we still use chemotherapy, although we use it in a way which I believe is more targeted and safer. We also embrace tools such as radiation and surgery, when indicated. It is important for people—particularly those who are more natural-minded—to remember that these are tested and proven methods for dealing with cancer. It makes little sense to abandon these therapies simply because they are not ideal or perfect, especially when dealing with a complex and aggressive disease such as cancer.

Surgery, in particular, is often a critical first step in treating cancer. Many patients come into my office having avoided surgery, even after a diagnosis of cancer, sometimes years prior. Many of these cases had remarkably good prognoses at the time of diagnosis, and still would were it not for patients delaying surgery indefinitely. Many people simply do not want to have surgery, for a variety of reasons including a fear of anesthesia, concerns over infection, and the belief that surgery spreads cancer.

Simply put, if a patient is a good candidate for surgery and the pros of a surgical procedure outweigh the cons, surgery is a critical first step in the treatment of cancer. An unwillingness to have surgery will likely make their journey much more difficult.

I am a firm believer in reviewing the conventional standard of care with any patient I see for consultation in my office. We discuss what the conventional approach would be based on the specifics of the diagnosis. I tell patients that we should consider these treatments as *part* of the plan. Some patients choose to take the purely conventional route, and if that is their choice, I always make the proper referrals. For some cancers which respond remarkably well to conventional treatment alone, I feel that this is a very reasonable choice.

For patients who choose to follow the integrative route, how we progress from that point differs dramatically from what a conventional protocol offers.

A Different Approach to Fighting Cancer

Integrative oncology sees the battle with cancer as having two fronts that must be addressed simultaneously. The first front is against a tumor (or, depending on the stage of disease, tumors). To this end, we have tools such as surgery to remove the tumor, and tools like chemotherapy and radiation which can shrink the tumor and/or kill cancer cells. Conventional oncology is well adept at fighting cancer in this regard.

Another front to the battle against cancer, however, is against the systemic burden of cancer. Cancerous tumors release what are called circulating tumor cells, or CTCs. A component of CTCs, known as cancer stem cells (or CSCs), can be thought of as synonymous for our purposes here. These cells are cancerous cells that can be found throughout the bloodstream, and are released by a tumor well before that tumor is able to be detected. Because of the nature of cancer cells, these cells are essentially immortal; they will not die unless we kill them, and they are floating around the body waiting on the right opportunity to form a tumor elsewhere. This spread from the primary site is known as metastasis.

Interestingly, conventional oncology largely ignores this systemic burden of cancer, especially in early stage cancers where the tumor is largely confined to one area. One of the biggest concerns with cancer is that even after successful treatment seemingly eliminates all traces of the disease, it can return years later. Because conventional oncology ignores these circulating tumor cells, we see that people can have surgery, full dose chemotherapy, and/or radiation, and be told they are "cancer-free," "cured," or "in remission," but get cancer again months or years later. In integrative oncology, we measure these levels of CTCs routinely, because they are critical for accurate diagnosis, appropriate treatment, and thorough monitoring. Many of the additional therapies we employ are aimed at killing these types of cells, as well as altering the "terrain" which provided an environment for cancer to grow and flourish.

Cancer as a Metabolic Disease

Another fundamental difference between integrative and conventional oncology is that integrative oncology treats cancer as a metabolic disease. Generally speaking, when we refer to metabolism, we are referring to how the body uses food to create energy. However, for our purposes, we need to think of metabolism on the cellular level; namely, the mechanisms by which cells obtain fuel and grow. At its core, treating cancer as a metabolic disease means that we attack the way cancer cells manufacture energy.

All cells—healthy cells and cancer cells—have a metabolic process by which they create energy. That energy currency is known as adenosine triphosphate, or ATP. Healthy cells produce upwards of 36 units of ATP as the result of their metabolic processes. You will recall that cancer cells have a very primitive way of producing energy that is heavily reliant on burning glucose, or sugar.

Also recall that one of the discoveries made by Dr. Otto Warburg nearly 100 years ago was that cancer cells thrive in a hypoxic—or oxygen deficient—environment. Hypoxia triggers something known as HIF-1 alpha, a gene which stimulates the production of glycolytic enzymes. These glycolytic enzymes mean that cancer cells are more dependent on glucose, which results in additional glucose receptors on the cell surface. These receptors are needed to bring glucose into the cell, which is then used to create energy. The result of cancer's inefficient energy creation process is only several units of ATP.

As opposed to the body's healthy cells, it seems that this is a very inefficient way of producing energy. However, when we think about the anabolic—or growth-producing—nature of cancer, this form of energy makes complete sense from a survival perspective. Regardless, it turns out that cancer prefers this method of energy, even when oxygen is in abundant supply. Because cancer cells are so reliant on glucose, they have more glucose and insulin receptors on their surface. We can use these characteristics of cancer cells to our advantage, in a variety of ways.

Another way we can use cancer's metabolic processes against it is by going after one of its primary metabolic byproducts, lactic acid. Cancer cells create an abundance of lactic acid as a result of their metabolism. This lactic acid can be thought of as a waste product. In order for a cancer cell to survive, that acid must be thrust out of the cell. Subsequently, we see that the areas surrounding cancer cells are far more acidic than the areas surrounding healthy cells. This is largely where you hear about the importance of pH in cancer development. We can use this in our favor. By targeting cancer's ability to remove lactic acid from the cells, and by targeting the acidic environment that surrounds cancer tumors and promotes their growth, we open ourselves up to more potentially effective treatment options.

Open-Minded Skepticism

While the methods used to diagnose and treat cancer today have a tremendous body of research which supports their use, there are many other methods used in integrative cancer treatment which have shown promise but have not been studied on the scale necessary to become mainstream. To ignore these types of studies is shortsighted in my opinion, especially given the fact that the outcomes from standard treatments have not significantly improved since President Nixon "declared war" on cancer nearly 50 years ago.

In evaluating potential treatments for my patients, I approach each one carefully, with open-minded skepticism. This is a philosophy I learned in my master's degree program in physiology at Georgetown University. As part of my degree program, in addition to courses in physiology and biochemistry, I took courses in complementary and alternative medicine. The objective of these courses was not merely to learn about various alternative therapies, but to learn how to evaluate scientific evidence for or against them. We were taught to neither accept nor reject a treatment at face value, but instead, to critically evaluate the evidence in order to make our own informed decisions. Through this process, I learned how to properly read scientific studies to look for bias as well as flaws in the study design. I still utilize those skills in my practice today, as potential "miracle" drugs, supplements, diets, and other treatments are introduced into the marketplace on a regular basis.

The paradigm of integrative oncology requires this open-minded skepticism. If a treatment has shown promise clinically and/or in a study, and if we believe that it could potentially provide benefit with a low likelihood of causing harm, why would we not at least consider its use? This approach should be contrasted with closed-minded skepticism, which is typically how conventional oncology views any cancer treatment outside of the standard of care, as well as open-minded acceptance, which is often how alternative medicine proponents view any natural treatment that has claims of effectiveness.

In integrative oncology, we seek to critically evaluate *all* potential therapies. This entails being open to their potential benefit, while also requiring that there be a solid scientific basis for how and why they work. For my practice, this has led to an interest in a variety of treatments and practices which I believe have greatly enriched my treatment protocols and outcomes.

A "Best of Both Worlds" Approach

The general principle behind integrative oncology is that we take the best aspects of modern medicine and the best aspects of natural medicine, and we combine these two philosophies in a strategic way so that the treatment protocol is personalized for each patient. We do not reject any treatment, unless we feel that the potential harms outweigh the potential benefits. Unfortunately, this reasonable approach is not common in cancer treatment today. Providers on both "sides" tend to embrace one philosophy while completely rejecting the other. This is neither evidence-based, nor is it fair to patients who are, many times, desperate for a comprehensive treatment program which addresses their treatment goals.

•———————————•

(1)   Lawenda, M.D. Brian D. "Hey Doc, Can I Take Antioxidants During Chemo and Radiation?" Integrative Oncology Essentials, 21 Mar. 2016, integrativeoncology-essentials.com/2013/03/hey-doc-can-i-take-antioxidants-during-chemo-and-radiation/. Accessed 15 Sept 2017.

(2)   Vetter ML, Herring SJ, et al. What do resident physicians know about nutrition? An evaluation of attitudes, self-perceived proficiency and knowledge. J Am Coll Nutr 2008; 27(2): 287-98.

(3)   Rossi RE, Pericleous M, Mandair D, et al. The role of dietary factors in prevention and progression of breast cancer. Anticancer Res 2014; 34(12): 6861-75.

(4)   Marshall JR. Diet and prostate cancer prevention. World J Urol 2012; 30(2): 157-65.

•———————————•

CHAPTER 4

Diagnostics

"Knowledge is power."
— Sir Francis Bacon

Cancer is a powerful adversary, and we should have as much information about it as possible if we seek to be victorious over it. This data can take on many forms, including blood testing, urine testing, saliva testing, imaging, and the often-forgotten physical exam. However, the first step is to obtain an accurate diagnosis, and this is done via a biopsy. After a biopsy confirms the presence of cancer, we must embark on a journey to obtain as much helpful information as possible. The more objective data we have at our disposal, the better.

Basic Lab Testing

Laboratory testing can provide us with a significant amount of information, and is ideally the first place to start after being diagnosed with cancer. My baseline lab panel, which is performed via blood testing, consists of a very thorough investigation into how the body is working. Below are some of the most important blood tests I order on my patients. Although all of these tests are readily available from most commercial labs, your oncologist will probably not be familiar with all of them.

Hopefully, your oncologist is open-minded and is thus willing to have a conversation with you. If so, I encourage you to ask him or her if you can have some of these tests which might not be part of their routine panel.

C-Reactive Protein

Often abbreviated as CRP, this lab test measures cellular inflammation, which is extremely important since we know that cancer is an inflammatory disease. Although cancer is not the only condition which can cause an increase in cellular inflammation, I have found that almost all cancer patients will have an elevated CRP. Striving to reduce CRP to more manageable levels should be one of the goals of treatment, since inflammation is not only consistent with cancer's presence, but also one factor used for its spread.

There are two C-reactive protein lab tests: CRP, and hsCRP (for high sensitivity C-reactive protein). The CRP measures inflammation of all cells in the body, whereas the hsCRP focuses more on the cells of the cardiovascular system. I prefer the CRP for cancer purposes.

As a side note, anyone interested in cardiovascular health, including prevention of heart attacks and strokes, should focus on hsCRP. This test has been shown to be a better predictor of cardiovascular disease risk than cholesterol.(1)

Ceruloplasmin

Ceruloplasmin is a liver protein that is responsible for storing and carrying copper throughout the body. Although the body needs some copper in order to carry out various processes, we do not want too much copper because cancer requires it for angiogenesis. Recall that angiogenesis is the formation of new blood vessels by cancer. The process of angiogenesis is a key component of cancer's growth and spread throughout the body.

Our goal ceruloplasmin when treating cancer is between 10 and 15 mg/dL, and of the many ceruloplasmin tests I have ordered, virtually no patients have met this goal on initial testing. Getting a handle on the ceruloplasmin level is a key component of any integrative cancer treatment program.

Complete Blood Count with Differential

This panel, often abbreviated as a CBC, is a standard panel ordered by almost all doctors, regardless of specialty. It provides important information about the body's cells, several of which are very important when dealing with cancer. This panel measures your white blood cell level, which is a key marker of general immune system function. Included in this panel are the different types of immune system cells, including neutrophils, lymphocytes, monocytes, eosinophils, and basophils. Each of these cells should be present in the body in specific amounts. Any abnormalities can signal an issue with the immune system, including a problem with the bone marrow where immune system cells are made.

The CBC also includes a measurement of the body's red blood cells, which are the oxygen-carrying cells of the body. Red blood cells also contain iron. In addition, this panel measures hemoglobin and hematocrit, both of which reflect the body's iron levels. Many cancer patients have low iron, which is reflected by low values here. As with the immune system cells, derangements here can signal an issue in the bone marrow where these cells are made.

Comprehensive Metabolic Panel

Often abbreviated as a CMP, the comprehensive metabolic panel evaluates key markers of the body's normal functioning. This panel includes a blood glucose (i.e., blood sugar) level, as well as markers of proper kidney and liver health. In addition, electrolytes including sodium and potassium are evaluated. This is a standard lab panel that most doctors will draw.

Of particular importance in this section is the albumin level. Albumin is a protein which is commonly used to evaluate liver health. However, it is also a marker of nutritional status, and many oncologists are unaware that decreases in albumin can signal a progression of cancer. Monitoring albumin to ensure that it stays optimized is key. Optimal is at least 4 g/dL. I routinely provide intravenous albumin to patients who have albumin levels below this optimal level.

Hemoglobin A1c

The hemoglobin A1c level provides valuable information about blood sugar control. In contrast to the blood glucose level, which is simply a blood sugar level at the time the blood was obtained, the hemoglobin A1c reflects the blood sugar over the previous three months. The hemoglobin A1c is the main way we diagnose type II diabetes today, because we know that diabetes is a disease of poor blood sugar control.

The higher the hemoglobin A1c level, the higher the blood sugar, and the poorer the patient's blood glucose control. We know that cancer loves sugar, and uses it as a preferred fuel source. Not surprisingly, having type II diabetes is associated with an increased risk of developing cancer. (2) However, simply avoiding the diagnosis of diabetes does not eliminate the risk for cancer. Interestingly, even those individuals in the high-normal hemoglobin A1c range have also been shown to be at increased risk of developing cancer. (3)

Although a hemoglobin A1c less than 5.7% is considered normal, an optimal hemoglobin A1c is 5% or less. I strive for this optimal range when I counsel my patients.

Hormones

There are many hormones in the body, and they each perform various functions. Having a firm understanding of how your hormones work is important, whether you have a type of cancer typically associated with hormones or not. Establishing a baseline level of hormones is especially important when dealing with those cancers which are frequently fueled by hormones, including breast, ovarian, and prostate.

For women, I typically check the main hormones, including estrogen (estradiol), progesterone, testosterone, and DHEA-S. For men, I check testosterone (free and total), estradiol, and DHEA-S. In addition, prolactin is a helpful hormone to check since it promotes growth of many cancers. Finally, checking a thyroid panel on both men and women provides a general look at overall metabolism. This panel should include thyroid stimulating hormone (TSH), free T4, free T3, and thyroid antibodies (TPO Ab and/or Thyroglobulin Ab).

Insulin-like Growth Factor 1

This lab test, also known as IGF-1, is a surrogate marker for growth hormone. Many cancers over-express IGF-1, meaning that we can use it to assess the extent of cancer in the body.

Iron Studies

We have already discussed the fact that iron can serve as fuel for cancer cells. Although the body needs some iron, we do not want too much. Iron studies evaluate the body's iron levels. This typically includes iron, total iron binding capacity, transferrin, transferrin saturation, and ferritin. Each of these measurements reflects iron in its different forms found inside the body. This complete panel of iron levels gives us valuable information as to the patient's overall iron status.

Chronic illnesses such as cancer can create a condition known as anemia of chronic disease. This frequently results in a high ferritin level, which is also a sign of inflammation. In addition, cancer patients can become anemic due to iron deficiency, which is usually treated with iron supplementation. I prefer to supplement with iron glycinate because it does not cause constipation like generic over-the-counter iron formulations. Intravenous iron, in the form of iron sucrose (Venofer), can be given for more severe anemias. Ultimately, we strive to treat the underlying source of the anemia so that it is not a continual problem.

Lactate Dehydrogenase

Frequently abbreviated as LDH, lactate dehydrogenase is another lab test which can be used to evaluate the extent of cancer. Although it is a non-specific test (i.e., it can be elevated in non-cancerous conditions as well), I have found that it is still helpful to measure when monitoring treatment progress. One study found that a high level of LDH in cancer patients corresponds to a greater risk of death. (4)

Lipid Panel

The lipid panel, also referred to as a cholesterol panel, is valued for its ability to evaluate heart health and cardiovascular disease risk. This panel includes total cholesterol, high-density lipoprotein (HDL), low-density lipoprotein (LDL), and triglycerides. Recommendations from many medical organizations over the past 50 years have consistently been for patients to aggressively lower their cholesterol. Interestingly, what most doctors do not know is that lower cholesterol is not usually better. Studies have shown that people with higher cholesterol actually live longer. (5) With respect to cancer, multiple studies have shown that cancer development is associated with low cholesterol, and that this can often precede the cancer diagnosis by decades. (6)

The reality is that what we have been told for decades about cholesterol is false. Sadly, most patients today still believe that cholesterol is bad, especially LDL cholesterol, and that cholesterol must be lowered as much as possible. This is despite evidence suggesting that even LDL, long referred to as "bad cholesterol," plays a role in proper immune system functioning. (7) Of course, this important function of LDL cholesterol is almost never shared with the public.

My approach to cholesterol levels in cancer is to neither allow them to get too high nor too low. A total cholesterol level between 200-250 is typically what I strive for in my patients. I also try to keep the LDL level under 160 or so, and the HDL over 50. These ranges are general ones, and obviously do not apply to every patient.

One additional note about cholesterol: I have found that patients with very low cholesterol tend to have very advanced cancer. Thus, I view very low cholesterol on lab testing as a poor prognostic sign, especially when the patient has longstanding cancer.

Lymphocyte Panel

Lymphocytes are key immune system cells, and measuring these individual cells provides us an important look at the immune system's functioning. The lymphocytes I recommend testing are CD3 T cells, CD4 T cells, CD8 T cells, and NK cells.

Tumor Markers

Most oncologists will order tumor markers on their patients. These markers are often, but not exclusively, released by cancer cells. Although they are not considered diagnostic, their presence can provide a way of monitoring response to treatment.

The main tumor markers are:

- AFP — a marker for liver, ovarian, and testicular cancers
- CA 125 — a marker for ovarian and breast cancers
- CA 15-3 — a marker for breast cancer
- CA 19-9 — a marker for gastrointestinal cancers
- CA 27.29 — a marker for breast cancer
- CEA — a marker for many types of malignancies, including breast, gastrointestinal, lung, and pancreatic cancers
- PSA — a marker for prostate cancer

When elevated above the normal range, they provide a meaningful number to track. When the number goes down, we assume that the cancer is responding to treatment. When the number goes up, the tendency is to assume that the cancer is worsening. However, tumor markers can also go up when cancer cells are dying as a result of treatment. In addition, many people with known cancer will have tumor markers in the normal ranges. Finally, there can be slight elevations in tumor markers due to non-cancerous conditions.

I measure applicable tumor markers on my patients, and monitor them routinely. However, it is irresponsible to put all of our confidence in these numbers since they are not 100% reliable.

Vitamin B12

This vitamin is important for a variety of important bodily processes, and many people supplement their diets with B12. However, elevated vitamin B12 levels have been associated with an increased risk of cancer. (8) This study evaluated B12 levels in patients without known cancer and who were not taking a B12 supplement. Interestingly, those with the highest B12 levels (> 600 pmol/L) had the highest risk of developing cancer. Most of these diagnoses were made within the first year of follow-up.

Most cancer cells have an over-expression of vitamin B12 receptors on their cell surface. (9) The same is also true for folate (vitamin B9) receptors. It is thought that cancer cells require more vitamin B12 and folate because these two vitamins are needed for rapid growth.

While it is neither feasible nor necessary to avoid vitamin B12 when battling cancer, I do feel that caution should be used when supplementing with B12. For those who are truly deficient in B12, it is reasonable to supplement the diet with it. However, for those who do not have B12 deficiency, supplementing with it—especially in mega-doses—is likely to be counterproductive and perhaps even dangerous.

Vitamin D

Vitamin D is a very important marker. We have long known that vitamin D is necessary for bone integrity, but research in recent years has revealed that vitamin D is also very important for proper immune system functioning. There is also research that vitamin D plays a protective role against heart disease and dementia.

The level of vitamin D to measure in the blood is called 25-OH vitamin D. Most labs consider a level below 30 ng/mL to be consistent with vitamin D deficiency. However, studies have shown that a level between 50-70 ng/mL should be our target when dealing with cancer. This level ensures that the immune system is appropriately stimulated.

In order to achieve a 25-OH vitamin D level of 50-70 ng/mL, supplementation will be required. It is not possible to get enough from the sun or consuming dairy. A high quality vitamin D supplement is essential.

Alternative Lab Testing

In addition to the blood tests mentioned above, there are some other tests which provide valuable information. Some of these tests are cancer-specific, while others are helpful in evaluating the body's functioning as a whole.

Cancer Profile

The Cancer Profile, or CA Profile to which it is commonly referred, is a lab panel developed by Dr. Emil K. Schandl of American Metabolic Laboratories in Hollywood, FL. This test requires both blood and urine specimens, and measures several markers thought to be associated with and/or elevated in cancer. These include phosphohexose isomerase (PHI) enzyme, human chorionic gonadotropin (HCG), and carcinoembryonic antigen (CEA).

As is the case with other alternative lab tests, the CA Profile is not part of the standard of care. However, it can be helpful in monitoring the cancer burden in the body as well as the patient's response to treatment.

Caris Molecular Intelligence

The Caris Molecular Intelligence test is an innovative test which analyzes a patient's tissue for specific genetic alterations. This is a very convenient test, as Caris obtains the tissue from a pathology lab which contains a patient's biopsy or surgical specimen. Once Caris receives the specimen, in-depth analysis is performed to evaluate the presence and activity level of hundreds of genes. Based on the results, treatment decisions can be made regarding which pharmaceutical agents might be most effective.

I especially like this test because it is backed by excellent, up-to-date research. It allows for the ultimate in personalized cancer treatment, which is especially important when we are dealing with pharmaceutical agents.

Circulating Tumor Cells

We know that cancer is not just a disease of the breast, colon, or prostate, but of the entire body. By the time a tumor is just several millimeters in size (much too small to be detected on a CT scan, PET scan, or MRI), it is already releasing what are known as circulating tumor cells into the blood. These circulating tumor cells, also known as CTCs, are cancer cells which ultimately lead to the progression and spread of cancer if not eliminated. Anyone who has had cancer—even someone who is in "remission"—will often have some level of CTCs. Thus, it is obvious that we should be measuring these cells, not only at the time a cancer diagnosis is made, but also at regular intervals during and even after treatment. (10)

There are several tests which measure circulating tumor cells. Unfortunately, they use different methodologies and most are of questionable reliability. Only one CTC test is FDA cleared, and that is the CELLSEARCH test. This test is readily available in the United States through most standard labs. It is approved to detect circulating tumor cells of breast, colorectal, and prostate origin. Those patients who are found to have some level of circulating tumor cells through this test have a worse prognosis.

Although the CELLSEARCH test is the only FDA cleared CTC test, I believe that the Biocept CTC test is the most accurate. Its advanced technology allows for a wide variety of CTCs to be measured, and thus provides the best evaluation of cancer's systemic burden inside the body. Biocept is located in California, and typically has a turnaround time of just one week for results.

There are other circulating tumor cell analyses performed by labs outside the United States. The most well-known of these is the "Greek test," developed by the Research Genetic Cancer Centre (R.G.C.C.) in Greece. The formal name of this test is Onconomics Plus. While it is not a diagnostic tool, the Onconomics Plus test can be used to analyze the number of circulating tumor cells. It uses a different methodology from the CELLSEARCH and Biocept CTC tests, so these results cannot be directly compared. However, the Onconomics Plus test takes it a step further. After measuring the number of circulating tumor cells, it analyzes these cells for a variety of genetic markers, and then performs sensitivity testing in the lab to determine which chemotherapy agents and nutritional supplements kill these cancer cells the best.

The Greek test is controversial in integrative oncology circles. Some providers feel that it is an excellent test, while others are suspicious as to its actual validity. Although I believe it is a good test, I do have concerns about its prognostic capabilities. Even though we are evaluating a patient's circulating tumor cells, and those cells' response to various treatments, how well do those lab results correspond to what actually happens inside the body? As we know, the body is a very complex environment—much more complex than what we can replicate inside a petri dish.

Cytometric Profiling

This innovative test, developed by Larry Weisenthal, MD, Ph.D., and conducted by the Wiesenthal Cancer Group, performs chemosensitivity testing on cancerous body tissues. The test requires live tissue, meaning that fresh tissue must be obtained via an invasive procedure such as biopsy, surgery, or ascites fluid. The fluid is analyzed in Dr. Weisenthal's lab to determine which pharmaceuticals are most effective at killing cancer.

This seems to be an extremely accurate test, and is likely the most accurate way to determine the best chemotherapy and immunotherapy agents for each patient. An independent study found that this testing is 90% accurate, which is very good. However, it has several drawbacks. One, it is quite expensive. The cost depends on how many pharmaceutical agents are tested, but the cost typically ranges from $2,500 to $8,000, which is the responsibility of the patient. Second, and perhaps even more difficult, is the fact that the specimen used for testing must be carefully obtained and thus arranged for ahead of time. This requires the cooperation of a surgeon or interventional radiologist, and involves him or her agreeing to comply with the specific rules and restrictions for specimen collection and preservation. Normal specimen collection and processing will not suffice, and if a tissue sample has already been collected and preserved in the hospital pathology lab, it is no longer usable by Dr. Weisenthal. Thus, patients who have already had a biopsy or surgery cannot have this testing without undergoing another procedure.

Once the specimen is sent to Dr. Weisenthal's lab in California, he personally performs the analysis of each specimen. A report is provided to the physician and patient, and the results help guide decision-making with regard to treatment.

IvyGene

The IvyGene test is a relatively new test which measures what is known as methylated DNA in the blood. The presence of methyl groups, which are a combination of a carbon and three hydrogens ($-CH_3$), at specific sites within the genome are consistent with cancer. The IvyGene test helps identify the presence of cancer, and also provides a quantitative measure of disease. An IvyGene score of 19 or below is considered normal, while a score of 20 or more is considered elevated.

Although the IvyGene test is not diagnostic in nature, I do feel that it can be a valuable test to obtain at regular intervals to assess treatment progress. The lab is located in West Lafayette, Indiana. Insurance does not cover the test.

Micronutrient Testing

The Micronutrient Test by SpectraCell Laboratories measures the function of 35 vitamins, minerals, antioxidants, and amino acids within white blood cells. In addition, antioxidant function as well as immune system function are assessed.

I like this test because it helps identify nutritional imbalances. We know that nutritional imbalance is quite common today, and by measuring these key nutrient levels in the body, we can correct any deficiencies and bring the body back into balance. Having the appropriate balance is critical for an optimally functioning immune system and efficient energy production by the body's cells.

SpectraCell Laboratories is located in Houston, Texas. The Micronutrient Test is sometimes covered by insurance.

Organic Acids Test

This urine test measures various organic acids; these are chemical compounds which result from cellular energy production. This "metabolic snapshot" includes over 70 markers, including bacterial overgrowth, the presence of yeast, vitamin and mineral levels, oxidative stress measurements, neurotransmitter levels, and information regarding immune system function.

There are several urine organic acid tests available, but my preference is the organic acid test by The Great Plains Laboratory. The test kit allows patients to collect their urine at home and send it directly to the lab in Kansas.

Salivary Cortisol

Cortisol is the body's main stress response hormone, playing a role in the body's "fight or flight" response. However, it is also involved in helping control blood sugar levels, reducing inflammation, and regulating metabolism. Cortisol is produced by the adrenal glands, which sit on top of the kidneys.

In today's stressed-out society, cortisol is released far more often, and in much greater amounts, than it should be. This results in unhealthy stress on the adrenal glands, which can affect energy levels, immune system function, and hormonal balance. Blood testing for cortisol does not allow us to detect small fluctuations in cortisol levels, but saliva testing does. The test is called a four-point salivary cortisol, which involves collecting saliva four times throughout the day.

I use the Temporal Adrenal Profile (TAP) from Diagnos-Techs lab in Washington. The patient is given a test kit, and collects saliva first thing in the morning, at noon, late afternoon, and at bedtime. The results are measured, and compared to healthy cortisol levels. I frequently see abnormal levels, indicating that there is some degree of adrenal stress. It is important to correct this adrenal imbalance so that the body can function as it is supposed to.

Imaging

As the saying goes, "A picture is worth a thousand words." There are various imaging modalities we can use to obtain precise information about cancer, including its location and severity. There is no perfect imaging method, and each has its own respective pros and cons.

Computed Tomography

Also known as a CT scan or CAT scan, this modality consists of passing multiple x-ray beams through an area of the body. CT scans can evaluate some organs, bony structures, and the brain. They provide better images than x-rays, but also expose the patient to a significantly greater amount of radiation.

Magnetic Resonance Imaging

More commonly referred to as an MRI, this imaging technology uses radio waves instead of x-rays. A magnetic field is used to create a detailed image of an area of the body. The brain, muscles, tendons, and even nerves can be evaluated by MRI. A significant advantage of MRIs is their lack of radiation exposure. They also result in very detailed images. However, they do take longer than x-rays and CT scans, and can be quite expensive. For this reason, many insurance companies will not pay for MRIs, and instead favor CT scans.

Mammography

Mammograms use x-rays to produce an image of the breasts. They can detect tumors in the breast, although they are much better at finding slow-growing or pre-cancerous lesions than fast-growing tumors. Although mammograms are relatively inexpensive compared to other imaging modalities, they do have limitations. Mammograms are not as accurate for women with large, dense, or fibrocystic breasts. They also compress the breasts, and I have concerns about this degree of trauma to the breast. Finally, they expose the patient to radiation.

Perhaps the most concerning aspect of mammograms is their high occurrence of false positives. This results in many unnecessary biopsies. However, mammography remains the gold standard in conventional medicine.

Positron Emission Tomography

Also known as a PET scan, this technology is considered a metabolic imaging tool. As a result of the radiation and contrast agents used, it evaluates a patient's unique biology and biochemistry. PET scans provide an accurate way of distinguishing cancerous tumors from non-cancerous tumors, and are the gold standard for imaging cancer in the body. When evaluating the extent of cancer in the body, we perform a PET scan using radio-labeled glucose, because we know that cancer cells take up glucose at a much higher rate than do normal cells.

Although PET scans expose patients to radiation, they are still about half the dose of radiation of a CT scan. They can also be quite expensive, resulting in insurance companies denying coverage in favor of a cheaper scan such as a CT scan.

Thermography

Thermography is an innovative imaging modality which uses a specialized infrared camera to detect heat patterns in an area of the body. Areas of increased heat, sometimes referred to as "hot spots," often correspond to increased inflammation and/or angiogenesis. Thermography can pinpoint exact areas of concern, and is very sensitive to fast-growing and/or aggressive tumors. It is also non-invasive, non-compressive, and does not involve any radiation.

Thermography has a far lower rate of false positive results compared to mammography. Although thermography is not perfect, it is safe and inexpensive. I am a firm believer in it, and hope that it will be more commonly used in years to come. I am confident that it would help save lives as by detecting cancerous and precancerous lesions sooner.

Ultrasound

Ultrasounds incorporate sound waves to create an image of a body area. Like MRIs, ultrasounds do not involve any radiation. They allow for visualization of some soft tissues, as well as breasts and liver. However, they do not allow for evaluation of bones or muscles, and are quite operator-dependent. Ultrasounds are inexpensive in comparison to CT scans, MRIs, and PET scans.

X-Ray

X-rays have been around for many years, and create simple images by passing x-ray beams through specific areas of the body. They are good for evaluating bony structures, and can detect some lung pathologies as well. While x-rays can detect cancer in some cases, they are not good at imaging soft tissues such as muscles and tendons. They are also not an appropriate imaging modality for many organs.

Advantages of x-rays are that they are fast, inexpensive, and subject the patient to a low level of radiation.

———————●———————

(1) Datta S, Iqbal Z, and Prasad KR. Comparison between serum hsCRP and LDL cholesterol for search of a better predictor for ischemic heart disease. Indian J Clin Biochem 2011; 26(2): 210-13.

(2) Vigneri P, Frasca F, Sciacca L, et al. Diabetes and cancer. Endocr Relat Cancer 2009; 16(4): 1103-23.

(3) Goto A, Noda M, Sawada N, et al. High hemoglobin A1c levels within the non-diabetic range are associated with the risk of all cancers. Int J Cancer 2016; 138(7): 1741-1753.

(4) Wulaningsih W, Holmberg L, Garmo H, et al. Serum lactate dehydrogenase and survival following cancer diagnosis. Br J Cancer 2015; 113(9): 1389-96.

(5) Hamazaki T, Okuyama H, Ogushi Y, et al. Towards a Paradigm Shift in Cholesterol Treatment. A Re-examination of the Cholesterol Issue in Japan: Abstracts. Ann Nutr Metab 2015; 66(supplement 4): 1-116.

(6) Ravnskov U, McCully KS, and Rosch PJ. The statin-low cholesterol-cancer conundrum. QJM 2012; 105(4): 383-8.

(7) Ravnskov U. High cholesterol may protect against infections and atherosclerosis. QJM 2003; 96(12): 927-34.

(8) Arendt JFB, Pedersen L, Nexo E, et al. Elevated plasma vitamin B12 levels as a marker for cancer: a population-based cohort study. J Natl Cancer Inst 2013; 105(23): 1799-1805.

(9) Waibel R, Treichler H, Schaefer NG, et al. New derivatives of vitamin B12 show preferential targeting of tumors. Cancer Res 2008; 68(8): 2904-11.

(10) Simoneau R. Utilizing circulating tumor cells to predict late recurrence. *Oncology Times* 2018; 40(3): 8,10.

CHAPTER 5

Treatments in Integrative Oncology

*"Innovation is taking two things that already exist and
putting them together in a new way."*
—Tom Freston

One hallmark of integrative oncology is a focus on having as many potential treatments at our disposal as possible. These treatments should address the scientific advances we have made in our understanding of how cancer forms, as well as how it grows and spreads. By employing open-minded skepticism, while maintaining our stance that science is our guide and not our god, we have a framework for a truly integrative approach which takes into account the unique needs of each patient.

Fractionated Chemotherapy

Chemotherapy is one of the most feared forms of medical treatment in existence, and not necessarily without reason. The side effects of chemotherapy are often as unpleasant as the cancer it is being used to fight. Even with the remarkable advances made in chemotherapy regimens, it remains one of the biggest fears when it comes to treating cancer.

It is important to remember that chemotherapy does not have to be a dirty word. Chemotherapy has mountains of evidence supporting its use, and unbeknownst to many people, a significant number of chemotherapy agents are made from naturally-occurring, plant-based substances. I regularly use chemotherapy in my practice, but the way we use it differs dramatically from conventional oncology.

A conventional oncologist will determine your chemotherapy dosage by calculating your height and weight. The result is what is known as maximum tolerated dose, or MTD. We also refer to this as full dose chemotherapy. This method came into prominence after childhood acute lymphoblastic leukemia (ALL) was successfully treated this way. (1) Since that time, it has been shown to be a consistently effective approach in a few other cancers, such as testicular cancer and Hodgkin lymphoma. However, these cancers are less complex and have significantly fewer mutations than most other cancers. Cancers such as breast, prostate, and colorectal do not respond nearly as consistently to full dose chemotherapy, and side effects can be significant. Scientists have been questioning the "more is better" approach to chemotherapy for quite some time. (2) In fact, it was nearly twenty years ago when several forward-thinking scientists began testing lower doses of chemotherapy, given more frequently than full dose regimens. (3)

In integrative oncology, we also perform the same calculation using your height and weight, but only administer about 10-30% of what a normal oncologist would. This is known as fractionated chemotherapy, and there are several distinct advantages to this approach.

With full dose chemotherapy, there is a large window of time between the administration of the initial treatment and the subsequent treatment. Typically, patients will receive treatment once every 1-3 weeks, depending on the chemotherapeutic agent(s) used, the type of cancer, and the stage of cancer. With this method, side effects frequently occur, including immune system suppression, nausea, vomiting, diarrhea, and fatigue. Administering full-dose chemotherapy more often than this would likely cause even more terrible side effects.

During that window of time between chemotherapy treatments, however, you give cancer cells that survived the treatment the opportunity to build resistance to the drug. We have learned that most tumors contain a proportion of cancer cells that are sensitive to treatments such as chemotherapy, while the remaining cancer cells are resistant to it. Maximum tolerated dose chemotherapy kills the sensitive cancer cells, leaving behind a population of resistant cells which are essentially unaffected by the chemotherapy. These resistant cells are then able to use nutrients and other factors to aggressively grow and thrive. This is why we often see a dramatic reduction in tumor size and cancer markers during the first cycle or two of MTD chemotherapy, but aggressive recurrence of the cancer in the months that follow. Unfortunately, the success seen in those early cycles is nearly impossible to maintain, as subsequent chemotherapy treatments against the remaining resistant cells provide little to no results.

A strategy which administers lower doses of chemotherapy more frequently has been developed. This is known as metronomic chemotherapy. (4) Because the dosage used each time with metronomic chemotherapy is less—or fractionated—the side effects are greatly mitigated if not non-existent, and the collateral damage to healthy cells is also greatly reduced. Another advantage of lower doses of chemotherapy given in this fashion is an anti-angiogenic effect, meaning that blood supply to the cancer is decreased. (5) Not surprisingly, such an approach was also found to greatly reduce toxicity. (6)

Insulin Potentiation Therapy (IPT)

In order to maximize the efficacy of fractionated chemotherapy, we take advantage of some of the metabolic properties of cancer. Recall that cancer cells have many more receptors for insulin and glucose on their cell membranes, because those cancer cells thrive on glucose, or sugar. This is the basis for insulin potentiation therapy—IPT.

Prior to administering chemotherapy, we lower the patient's blood sugar by administering insulin; typically, we try to lower the patient's blood sugar to between 35-55 mg/dL. This creates what we call a therapeutic moment, the point at which we believe cancer cells become desperate for glucose. It is at this point where we administer intravenous glucose, known as dextrose, along with multiple chemotherapeutic agents strategically and carefully chosen for that patient based on advanced testing. By bringing the patient's blood sugar back up, while at the same time administering chemotherapy, we believe we can better target the chemotherapy drugs directly toward cancerous cells. In this way, lower dosages of chemotherapy become more like a heat-seeking missile than an atom bomb.

In addition to being more targeted toward cancer, fractionated chemotherapy has the added benefit of stimulating immune response. It has also been shown to reduce angiogenesis, or the creation of new blood vessels to feed cancer tumors. These are not benefits typically seen in full-dose chemotherapy, which as we all know, often wrecks the immune system, harms the body's healthy cells, and creates resistant cancer cells.

The challenge with fractionated chemotherapy using IPT is that we do not have large-scale clinical trials evaluating its efficacy. This is not surprising, as studies involving many patients treated for years require significant funding, and this funding most often comes from pharmaceutical companies. Pharmaceutical companies have little incentive to investigate the possibility that their drugs work just as well, if not better, using 1/10th to 1/3rd of the usual doses. An ideal study would compare full dose chemotherapy, given the usual way, with fractionated chemotherapy, administered with IPT.

Although fractionated chemotherapy and IPT are not yet the standard of care, they are not new concepts. IPT was first developed in the 1930s in Mexico by Dr. Donato Perez Garcia. He theorized that insulin could improve the cellular uptake of other medications given, since insulin was already known at that time to be required for the uptake of sugar. For the first couple of decades, Dr. Garcia treated several different diseases using IPT, including schizophrenia and syphilis. It was not until later that he began using IPT to treat cancer in conjunction with low dose (or fractionated) chemotherapy. Today, IPT is primarily used for cancer treatment at a select group of cancer treatment clinics, as mainstream cancer treatment centers only administer treatments considered that are considered within the standard of care.

Despite a lack of long-term, randomized, placebo-controlled trials involving fractionated chemotherapy given with IPT, there are some studies which shed light on how it works. The current belief is that IPT affects the metabolism of cancer cells, making them more sensitive to chemotherapy agents (thus the reason for using significantly less chemotherapy). It is also believed that the insulin and glucose given in conjunction with chemotherapy better target the chemotherapy to the cancer cells, rather than healthy cells. (7) This is consistent with previous research confirming that cancer cells have significantly more insulin and glucose receptors on their cell surface compared to healthy cells.

Although it would be wonderful to be able to conduct long-term clinical trials on fractionated chemotherapy with IPT, this is unlikely to occur. As mentioned previously, there is little incentive for a pharmaceutical company to pay for a study on a drug which would possibly result in an 80-90% reduction in the current doses used. This would greatly cut into their profits. I am not a conspiracy theorist by any means, but it is important to remember that pharmaceutical companies are businesses which strive to make profits for themselves and their shareholders. If a drug company is not going to fund a large-scale study, we unfortunately are not left with many options.

Fractionated chemotherapy administered with IPT makes sense to me on a biochemical and physiological level. Despite it not being "proven," I have seen it work very well in my own practice with my patients. It is a much safer way to administer chemotherapy in many cases, and I believe it is efficacious, as well. I do not think it is appropriate for everyone, but for those patients who have either failed full dose chemotherapy previously, are not candidates for full dose chemotherapy, or who prefer to try a gentler and safer approach, it is an excellent tool in our toolbox.

Off-Label Use of Pharmaceuticals

The way we use insulin with chemotherapy is considered an "off-label" use of insulin, a drug that is approved for treating diabetics. Off-label use of pharmaceuticals is viewed by physicians as an acceptable choice when there is scientific evidence supporting a drug's potential benefit, coupled with a low likelihood of causing harm. However, this has not become a common occurrence in conventional oncology, in spite of the fact that there is solid evidence suggesting that many drugs can be effectively repurposed to fight cancer.

This, too, is shortsighted. If we think that drugs which have already been tested for safety, whose contraindications we are already aware of, might show some promise for fighting cancer, why would we not repurpose those drugs for that use? That would be like members of the Manhattan Project saying that nuclear fission was created only for use as a weapon; we should not repurpose it as a method for creating energy. Yet, this illogical thought process is pervasive in medicine, and particularly in oncology. Why would we not try to take advantage of their anti-cancer effects in a clinical setting, provided they are used in a safe and responsible way under the care of a skilled physician?

It turns out that insulin is just one of the drugs we can use "off-label" for treating cancer. A 2012 research paper, entitled "Hiding in Plain View," investigated many existing pharmaceuticals for an anti-cancer effect. Not surprisingly, they found many promising candidates. One quote from the authors was especially striking: "We advocate that confirmation of these findings in randomized trials be considered a high research priority, as the potential impact on human lives saved could be immense." (8)

I share their enthusiasm regarding the value in off-label pharmaceuticals for the treatment of cancer. As you will see, many of these medications have been shown to pack a powerful anti-cancer punch, while having little to no apparent side effects or safety concerns.

Metformin

Metformin (glucophage), a drug approved as first-line treatment of type 2 diabetes, is another drug that we use off-label. However, an interesting finding occurred over the years in studying Metformin: diabetics who took Metformin were found to have a 54% lower risk of developing cancer compared to diabetics not taking Metformin. (9) There are several mechanisms for Metformin's anti-cancer effect, the most prominent of which is its inhibition of what is known as the mammalian target of rapamycin (mTOR) pathway. (10) We know that the mTOR pathway is a major player in cancer cell growth, spread, and survival. (11) If we can disrupt the mTOR pathway, we stand a much greater chance of slowing down cancer.

In addition, Metformin is thought to target cancer by reducing the available insulin and insulin-like growth factor 1 (IGF-1), both of which are heavily utilized by cancer cells. (12) Finally, Metformin has been shown in multiple studies to kill cancer stem cells, which can be thought of as a subset of circulating tumor cells, known as CTCs. (Often, the terms "cancer stem cell" and "circulating tumor cell" are used interchangeably.) Addressing circulating tumor cells in the blood is a critical tool for reducing the chances of metastases in the future.

Metformin is a very safe medication, but it does cause gastrointestinal upset in approximately 25-30% of patients. However, this side effect is greatly reduced when using the extended-release form. Because Metformin works with the body's physiology, rather than apart from it, the chances of hypoglycemia (low blood sugar) are extremely rare. Nonetheless, it is a prescription and should be monitored by a cancer physician who is familiar with its use in this setting.

Ammonium Tetrathiomolybdate

One of the drugs I am most excited about as an anti-cancer agent is ammonium tetrathiomolybdate, called TM for short. I was introduced to ammonium tetrathiomolybdate by Mark Rosenberg, MD, an integrative oncologist in Boca Raton, FL and also a mentor of mine. TM is a drug initially developed to treat Wilson's disease, a disorder where excess copper accumulates in the body. The body needs some copper, but excess copper as seen in Wilson's disease causes significant problems unless it is chelated. Chelation of a substance, such as a metal, allows it to be appropriately eliminated from the body. As we see with many drugs, the patent on ammonium tetrathiomolybdate ran out and newer drugs were created which supplanted it. The result is that TM was mostly forgotten about.

However, research has since uncovered the role of copper in angiogenesis—the formation of new blood vessels to supply cancer with nutrients and other resources needed for it to grow. Recall that angiogenesis is one of the hallmarks of cancer discussed previously. It turns out that copper is required for angiogenesis, and if we reduce the amount of copper available in the body, cancer will be deprived of a very important substrate. In addition to lowering copper, TM also reduces blood levels of other substances needed by cancer to grow, including vascular endothelial growth factor (VEGF), fibroblast growth factor (FGF), interleukin-6 (IL-6), and interleukin-8 (IL-8). (13) There are also studies suggesting that TM improves the effectiveness of various chemotherapy agents.

In my practice, I routinely check a blood level of copper, known as ceruloplasmin, on every patient. I have found that ceruloplasmin is almost always elevated, or at least in the high-normal range, when cancer is present. The use of ammonium tetrathiomolybdate as an off-label agent in cancer, with the express purpose of chelating copper, allows us to reduce copper to a much safer level. The "sweet spot" is a copper level low enough that we are preventing or greatly reducing angiogenesis, but not quite to zero since the body does need some copper for normal cellular processes.

I have found ammonium tetrathiomolybdate to be an extremely valuable tool. It is my belief that most everyone with cancer should be on it. Because it is no longer commercially available, it must be compounded by a compounding pharmacy with expertise in it. Since it is also a weak chelator of iron, iron levels in the body should be monitored regularly. However, it is a very safe and well-tolerated drug. It is typically continued for up to 3 years.

Itraconazole

This anti-fungal drug, commonly used to treat a wide variety of fungal infections in the body, has been shown to have an anti-cancer effect. It might seem paradoxical that a drug used to treat fungus can also target cancer. However, the link between cancer and fungus is not new. Doug Kaufmann, a friend and colleague of mine, and host of the nationally syndicated television show, Know the Cause, is an expert on fungus and its effects on our health. His hypothesis that fungi, and their secondary byproducts known as mycotoxins, can induce DNA damage and thus cause cancer is supported by numerous studies. (14, 15)

Moreover, the similarities between fungi and cancer cannot be ignored. Both thrive on sugar as an energy (ATP) source, both produce ATP in the absence of oxygen, and both accumulate lactic acid. Is it really surprising, then, that anti-fungal drugs have been found to have an anti-cancer effect in studies?

In a study on males with advanced prostate cancer, itraconazole was found to have modest anti-cancer activity. (16) Studies in other types of cancer have been encouraging as well. Because it is an anti-fungal drug, we must be intentional about protecting gut health. Antifungal agents can inadvertently kill the good bacteria in the digestive tract, so a focus on providing beneficial gut bacteria through diet and supplementation is imperative.

In addition, we must address sources of fungus in our lives. Although edible mushrooms are fungi, and limiting or avoiding them altogether is recommended, we are also incidentally exposed to mycotoxins through other foods in our diets as well as elsewhere in our environment.

Doxycycline

This antibiotic has been used for over 50 years to treat a wide variety of bacterial infections, but it has also been shown in multiple studies to have several anti-cancer effects. First, it inhibits a key group of enzymes known as matrix metalloproteinases (MMPs) (17), which are responsible for cancer growth and spread. Second, doxycycline has been shown to kill cancer stem cells while also being synergistic with IV vitamin C. (18) Finally, doxycycline makes these CSCs more susceptible to damage to radiation therapy. (19)

As with antifungal agents, antibacterial agents can deplete beneficial bacteria in the gut, so a robust probiotic supplement is in order.

Cimetidine

Cimetidine, also known as Tagamet, is a drug commonly used to treat gastroesophageal reflux disease (GERD) as well as peptic ulcers. It blocks one of the histamine receptors known as H2. However, it has been shown to have anti-tumor activity in the treatment of colorectal cancer (20), kidney cancer (21), and melanoma. (22) Studies have found that it helps maintain lymphocyte counts and natural killer (NK) cell counts, both of which are important markers of immune system activity. (23)

Cimetidine can inhibit the action of other drugs, so great care must be taken when considering its use as part of an integrative protocol.

Rapamycin

Rapamycin is a natural substance produced by the bacteria Streptomyces hygroscopicus, first isolated on Easter Island in the southeastern Pacific Ocean in the early 1970s. It was originally used as an anti-fungal compound, due to its ability to affect a component of yeast known as target of rapamycin (TOR). It was later found to suppress the immune system in humans, as TOR is also found in mammalian cells. (24) In humans, we call this mTOR, which stands for mammalian target of rapamycin. We know that mTOR is responsible for many key cellular functions, such as growth and energy production. It can be thought of as the gas pedal which causes the cell to "go." Thus, it is a necessary component of healthy cells.

Unfortunately, mTOR is almost always "hijacked" by cancer cells. In fact, mTOR is responsible for the aggressive growth we see in cancer cells. Rapamycin is of interest to us in treating cancer because it decreases mTOR. However, we must strike a balance here since too much rapamycin will suppress the immune system. Thankfully, including grapefruit with rapamycin improves the bioavailability of rapamycin. This means that we can use about half of the rapamycin dose to achieve the same effectiveness, while also greatly reducing toxicity. An 8 ounce glass of grapefruit juice has been shown to increase rapamycin levels by 350%! (25)

Any concerns about potential immunosuppression when using rapamycin in cancer treatment were addressed in a 2004 study, which found that the drug's anti-cancer activities are dominant over its immunosuppressant effects. (26)

Noscapine

This naturally occurring component of the poppy family is commonly used for its antitussive effect. It has been shown to have an anti-cancer effect as well. One study found that it inhibited cancer while producing little to no toxicity, including no damaging effects to the immune system response. (27) It was also found to inhibit what is known as hypoxia-inducible factor-1 (HIF-1), a component of tumors which is correlated with advanced disease and poor prognosis. (28) It stands to reason that inhibiting HIF-1 could significantly improve life span as well as quality of life in cancer patients.

Noscapine is well absorbed in its oral form, seems to work well with other treatments, has low toxicity, and is low-cost. As is true for several other older drugs which we are repurposing for cancer treatment, noscapine must be made by a compounding pharmacy.

Disulfiram (Antabuse)

This medication was developed in the 1920s to treat alcoholism. When alcohol is ingested, it must be broken down by the liver, and a key enzyme in this process is known as acetaldehyde dehydrogenase. Disulfiram inhibits this enzyme, and as a result, causes severe hangover symptoms when someone taking disulfiram drinks alcohol. As with many drugs, it was very popular for a period of time and then fell out of favor as newer drugs were developed and patented.

Disulfiram's anti-cancer activity is significant; it directly causes apoptosis (cell death) of many different types of cancer cells. It also inhibits a component of cancer cells known as nuclear factor kappa B (NF-kB). In a cancer cell, NF-kB is a pathway which controls cancer growth and development. By inhibiting NF-kB, disulfiram is decidedly anti-cancer. Studies have shown that it has anti-tumor, anti-metastatic, and anti-angiogenic properties against cancer cells, and that it does so at non-toxic doses. (29)

Not surprisingly, alcohol must be avoided entirely when taking disulfiram, even at doses used for anti-cancer purposes. Even herbal tinctures made with very small amounts of alcohol should be excluded from the protocol, as reactions with disulfiram will still occur. If the tincture is an essential component of the protocol, the alcohol will need to be boiled off before ingesting.

Dipyridamole (Persantine)

This agent is known for opposing platelets, which are a component of blood clotting. We typically think of it as being used for preventing blood clots in patients prone to heart attacks and strokes. However, it can be beneficial in the treatment of cancer, as well.

Elevated platelets are often seen in cancer patients. This is a troubling finding, because platelets are known to reflect inflammation. This situation recruits growth factors, which cancer uses to spread. Elevated platelets also increase risk of blood clots, which is one reason why cancer patients have more clots than non-cancer patients. Thus, blocking platelets can have a powerful anti-cancer effect.

There have been some very encouraging studies involving dipyridamole. One particularly notable study looked at pancreatic cancer patients receiving dipyridamole along with the standard of care chemotherapy regimen (5-fluorouracil, leucovorin, and mitomycin). These pancreatic cancer patients were not surgical candidates, meaning that they had a very poor prognosis with a predicted survival of approximately 8-12 months. In the 38 patients studied, 70% survived one year and 27% of these patients were able to undergo surgery to remove the cancer. These patients had a one-year survival rate of 83%, far superior to the conventional standard. (30) The significant improvement in survival was appropriately attributed to the dipyridamole, as it was the only agent which was added to the usual treatment regimen.

Clarithromycin (Biaxin)

This antibiotic is part of a class of drugs known as macrolide antibiotics. Clarithromycin is used to treat infections, especially those of the sinuses, lungs, and gastrointestinal tract. It is also a treatment for Lyme disease. It has been shown in the years since it was first discovered to also have several notable anti-cancer properties, including the inhibition of nuclear factor kappa beta (NF-kB) and suppression of tumor necrosis factor alpha (TNF-alpha). Clarithromycin is anti-angiogenic (31), and has also been shown to reduce cachexia. Cachexia is the wasting syndrome we see in advanced cancers, involving loss of appetite, fatigue, weight loss, and muscle atrophy.

The sum total of the research on clarithromycin is consistent with a significant survival benefit. In a study of 49 patients with inoperable lung cancer, those receiving clarithromycin survived twice as long on average compared to those patients who did not. There were no notable side effects noted in the study. (32)

Naltrexone

This drug was developed over 30 years ago to assist patients in overcoming drug addiction. By blocking the opioid receptor, the addiction potential of the drug is reduced. A secondary effect of blocking the opioid receptor is also an inhibition of beta-endorphin and metenkephalin; this inhibitory action boosts the immune system. It has since been determined that we can achieve these powerful immune-boosting effects with much lower doses of naltrexone (approximately 1/10th of the dose used for combating addiction). We refer to this as low dose naltrexone, or LDN.

From an anti-cancer perspective, the benefit of low dose naltrexone seems to be an increase in the number of natural killer cells as well as their activity. (33) Natural killer cells are important components of the immune system response, and are often deficient in cancer.

I feel that LDN has a lot of potential. It is typically taken at bedtime, as the immune system is especially active when we are sleeping. It must be compounded by a compounding pharmacy, but is inexpensive. It also seems to be very safe, with the only known side effect being vivid dreams.

Aspirin

Aspirin, also known as acetylsalicylic acid (ASA), is derived from willow bark. It is rumored that Hippocrates, the father of modern medicine, had his patients chew on bark from the willow tree to help bring a fever down. The cardiovascular benefits from daily aspirin are well documented.

In addition to its effect on heart health, it has long been known that those who take aspirin have a lower incidence of cancer compared to those who do not. This is especially true in the prevention of colorectal cancer, as evidenced by a study showing that those taking a daily aspirin had a 24% reduction in risk of developing colorectal cancer. This benefit was only apparent after taking aspirin for 5 years. (34)

But what about aspirin as a cancer treatment, when we already have a cancer diagnosis? A recent study evaluated all existing evidence for low dose aspirin in the treatment of cancer, and concluded that it could increase survival by up to 20% and significantly reduce metastases. (35)

The decision regarding whether to add aspirin to the protocol is one that should not be taken lightly, as it is a blood thinner which can interact with other medications. Nonetheless, for a large majority of patients, it is extremely well-tolerated and is an excellent candidate for inclusion in an anti-cancer protocol.

Propranolol

Propranolol is a drug used to treat high blood pressure. It is in a class of antihypertensive medications known as beta blockers, due to its activity against what are known as beta-adrenergic receptors. These receptors are a component of the sympathetic nervous system, which governs our body's "fight or flight" response. By blocking these beta-adrenergic receptors, beta blockers lower blood pressure.

However, propranolol—as well as several other beta blockers—have been shown to have an anti-cancer effect. Epidemiological studies on men taking drugs for high blood pressure found that those taking beta blockers had a lower risk of developing prostate cancer. (36) Further studies found that cancer patients taking a beta blocker have a lower risk of cancer death. (37)

This brings up a very important point regarding the link between stress, cancer development, and cancer death. Why would a blood pressure drug reduce both cancer development and cancer death? The answer lies in the mechanism of how these drugs work in the body. By reducing the "fight or flight" portion of the nervous system, the stress—or perceived stress—on the body is greatly reduced. This reinforces our long-held belief that stress plays a role in cancer. In fact, a recent study confirmed that stress-induced activation of the neuroendocrine system resulted in a 30-fold increase in cancer spread. (38)

Because we all have stress in our lives, we must take great care to reduce our stress as much as possible in order to lower our risk of developing cancer. Daily stress reduction practices such as prayer, meditation, laughter, and spending time with those we love are crucial, not only for our overall happiness, but also for our overall health. For those who are already dealing with a cancer diagnosis, stress is understandably very high, and reducing stress becomes even more important. In my integrative oncology practice, an emphasis on stress identification as well as stress reduction starts on day one of my treatment protocols.

Statins

Statin drugs are well known for their ability to lower cholesterol, although they have come under scrutiny in recent years due to their side effects as well as the fact that they also increase risk for developing type 2 diabetes. From a cardiovascular perspective, I feel that statins have been overprescribed. However, from a cancer perspective, they have a lot to offer in certain situations.

There are several effects of statins which are of interest to us in fighting cancer, including their ability to reduce inflammation, enhance the immune system, and oppose angiogenesis. One study found that people taking statins had a 47% reduction in their risk for developing colorectal cancer. (39) Another study examining statins and lung cancer risk found that those taking statins for at least 6 months had a 55% reduction in their risk of developing lung cancer. (40) The role of statins in prevention of cancer does not stop there, as patients who take statins seem to also have a lower risk of developing prostate cancer. (41)

What about using statins in patients already diagnosed with cancer? One study found that patients with liver cancer who were not surgical candidates, but who took a statin, survived twice as long as liver cancer patients who did not take a statin. (42) Statins also seem to be helpful in patients diagnosed with prostate cancer. A recent study in men with prostate cancer who had surgical removal of the prostate found that those who took a statin had a 30% lower chance of having their cancer recur. Men who took the highest doses of statins had even better results, a 50% lower chance of recurrence. (43)

The decision regarding statin use must be weighed carefully. The anti-cancer effect of statins is likely due to their ability to reduce inflammation and decrease the production of new blood vessels to feed cancer. However, statins also lower cholesterol, which is not necessarily a positive since cholesterol is needed to form cell membranes and also produce hormones in the body. In addition, the fact that statins increase the risk of developing type 2 diabetes is problematic, especially since poor blood sugar control is quite disadvantageous when treating cancer.

Patients often ask me if it is okay to use red yeast rice instead of statins. Red yeast rice is the natural supplement form of statins, and is thought to be safer. I am optimistic that this could be a wonderful solution, as red yeast rice does not cause the muscle aches that statins often do. Unfortunately, we do not have good studies examining the potential role of red yeast rice as an anti-cancer agent. I am hopeful that we will eventually see the same cancer treatment effect clinically with red yeast rice as we do statins.

pH Manipulation Therapy

At the cellular level, cancer behaves in a very characteristic fashion. Although science today focuses on cancer genetics, I believe that we should go farther upstream if we hope to be successful in our fight against cancer. While genes are certainly important, the genetic changes we see in cancer are a symptom rather than a cause. The true cause of cancer lies in its metabolism, or the way it makes energy. If we can disrupt the energy creation process, then we attack cancer at its core.

Cancer cell metabolism is actually quite primitive, and compares more favorably to lower life forms than it does healthy human cells. One characteristic of most cancer cells is that they preferentially use glucose (sugar) to make their energy through a process known as glycolysis. Healthy cells in the body use glycolysis as well, but then progress on toward a much more complex and elaborate mechanism to produce energy. Much of the energy production in healthy cells occurs in the mitochondria. In contrast, cancer cells have poorly functioning mitochondria, and thus stop after glycolysis, which is also known as fermentation. We term these cancer cells glycolytic. This is the basis for PET scans, which use radio-labeled glucose to show the presence of cancer. The more a tumor lights up on a PET scan, the more glycolytic it is.

The lactic acid produced by cancer cells is a waste product, formed as a consequence of making energy. This lactic acid must be released from the cancer cell in order for the cell to survive. The result of this efflux of acid is a higher, or more alkaline, pH inside the cancer cell and a lower, more acidic, pH in the space around the cancer cell, known as the extracellular space. In addition to allowing the cancer cell to survive, the acid excreted outside the cell also serves to fuel the progression of cancer in a few, specific ways. First, the acidic extracellular environment promotes metastasis. (44) It also works to neutralize certain chemotherapy drugs. It even inhibits the immune system. (45) Finally, it serves as a fuel source for other cancer cells.

As you can see, this pH issue is a very real problem when it comes to cancer, and we must address it if we hope to have consistent success against cancer. It is my belief that our failure to do so is a major reason why we have not seen much improvement in the cancer death rate over the past 50 years.

It turns out that there are several mechanisms by which cancer cells release lactic acid. The first is the sodium-hydrogen (Na-H) exchanger, which brings sodium into the cancer cell in exchange for releasing a hydrogen (acid) outside the cell. This is why we see lower sodium levels in the blood of advanced cancer patients. Another is the vacuolar-type hydrogen ATPase (V-type H+ ATPase), an enzyme which pumps acid outside the cell. There is also carbonic anhydrase 9 (CAIX), an enzyme which brings a bicarbonate ion into the cell in order to release acid outside the cell, and there is monocarboxylate 4 (MCT4), a transporter which releases lactate outside the cell.

Pharmaceutical research has shown us that the above processes can be inhibited. It is important to note that no medications have been created or approved for this use, so all of the uses for the medications that follow are considered off-label use. The off-label use of pharmaceutical agents is a common practice in medicine, but must be used with caution since any agent with a known action (pharmaceutical, natural supplement, or any other treatment) also has the potential for adverse reactions and side effects. We must weigh our oath to "first, do no harm" with our desire to attack cancer as aggressively and intelligently as possible.

With that said, we target the aforementioned acid pumps as follows:
- The sodium-hydrogen exchanger is inhibited by amiloride, a drug approved for treatment of heart failure and hypertension.
- Vacuolar-type hydrogen ATPase, which is inhibited by Prilosec (omeprazole), a medication approved for treatment of gastroesophageal reflux disease (GERD). Long-term use of proton pump inhibitors such as omeprazole can decrease magnesium levels in the body, known as hypomagnesemia. Thus, supplementation with a high quality, well-absorbed magnesium is essential in these situations.
- Carbonic anhydrase 9 is inhibited by acetazolamide, a drug approved for the treatment of glaucoma and altitude sickness.
- Monocarboxylate is inhibited by non-steroidal anti-inflammatory drugs (NSAIDs). I recommend Celebrex (celecoxib), which

has shown anti-cancer benefit in several studies by blocking cyclooxygenase-2 (COX-2), which we know is highly active in cancer. It also acts as an anti-inflammatory agent, which is important since we know that cancer is a highly inflammatory condition. In fact, Celebrex selectively affects DNA in cancer cells but not normal tissues. (46) Moreover, Celebrex has been shown to be effective in relieving cancer-related pain, especially when that pain is due to bone metastases.

The benefits of Celebrex in the treatment of cancer do not stop there. Celebrex enhances the effect of chemotherapy. (47) It has also been shown to be synergistic with several natural compounds, including curcumin (48) and green tea extract. (49)

The sum total of the therapies in this protocol is an inhibition of the release, or efflux, of acid from cancer cells. These treatments are intended for long-term use as long as we are fighting cancer. Some of these medications will require routine monitoring of kidney function, liver function, electrolytes, platelet counts, blood pressure, and other parameters.

It should be noted that the above protocol is not appropriate for all patients, as there are contraindications for their use in some situations. However, when possible, I feel that the above regimen can serve as an extremely powerful weapon in our cancer-fighting arsenal.

What About Alkaline Diets?

A natural follow-up question I receive after reviewing the above approach with patients involves an alkaline diet. The idea behind an alkaline diet is to address the acidity of cancer by eating specific foods with a higher pH to act as a buffer, thus making the body less acidic. We know that the pH scale goes from 0 to 14, with 0-7 being acidic and 7-14 being alkaline. A value of 7 is considered neutral, with the body's normal pH being at or around 7.4. The theory is that disease thrives in an acidic environment, and cannot exist in an alkaline environment. Generally speaking, the pH of foods is as follows: Vegetables, fruits, nuts, and legumes are thought to be alkaline. Animal proteins, dairy, and grains are thought to be acidic. Starches and sugars are thought to be neutral.

Many proponents of alkaline diets recommend focusing on alkaline foods, then testing the pH of urine and/or saliva to determine the body's pH. My personal belief is that this approach is an exercise in futility, as one of the primary jobs of the kidneys is to buffer the body's pH within a fairly narrow range. If you eat something acidic, such as chicken, your urine will be more acidic because the kidneys will excrete the excess acid. Likewise, if you eat something alkaline, the urine will soon be more alkaline because the kidneys are doing their job. The body is always monitoring and adjusting in order to keep the overall blood pH fairly stable, in the 7.35-7.45 range. Neither urine nor saliva are meaningful ways to measure the body's pH.

Besides, we must keep in mind that there is no such thing as an acidic body or an alkaline body. The pH inside the body varies greatly from one part to the next. For example, the stomach is very acidic, because that acidity is needed to properly digest the food we eat. As we move farther down the digestive tract, the pH becomes more alkaline, because the harsh acidity of the stomach would not be beneficial there. Our concern is to manipulate the pH in and around cancer cells, and we do that using the aforementioned protocol of off-label medications. There is no evidence that we can accomplish that through the foods we eat. I suspect that any benefits seen with an alkaline diet are due to the fact that alkaline foods are largely unprocessed, plant-based foods.

The ReDO Project

We often say when discussing treatments outside of mainstream medicine that, "more research is needed." Thankfully, there is a diverse group of physicians, scientists, and patient advocates who are researching existing non-cancer drugs in the hope that new, effective, and low-cost cancer treatments will be discovered. This is known as the Repurposing Drugs in Oncology (ReDO) Project, and the goal is to use these drugs in off-label fashion to supplement existing cancer treatments, or perhaps even develop entirely new treatment regimens altogether. They are currently researching a handful of drugs, and this is the kind of enterprising, outside-the-box thinking we need more of in cancer treatment today.

High-Dose Intravenous Vitamin C

Vitamin C has a variety of uses when it comes to cancer treatment. Vitamin C is an important antioxidant that is a key part of a healthy diet, but for the purposes of cancer treatment, the dosages required to obtain an anti-cancer effect must be administered intravenously. (50) There is a limit to how much vitamin C can be absorbed through the digestive system. This is not to say that oral vitamin C is not beneficial, but in terms of how we use it to fight cancer, administering vitamin C through an IV is necessary.

Research from over 40 years ago uncovered a potential benefit from high dose vitamin C. (51) Because of these encouraging results, a larger-scale trial was performed at the Mayo Clinic. This was a double-blind study of 100 patients with advanced colorectal cancer, none of whom had received chemotherapy. Those receiving vitamin C therapy were not found to have any objective improvement over those who did not. These results were published in the New England Journal of Medicine in 1985. (52) Not surprisingly, this study was used to conclude that IV vitamin C was not effective against cancer. However, this study used high dose oral vitamin C, and not intravenous vitamin C. This is significant, as we know that we can achieve much higher doses using IV vitamin C compared to oral vitamin C, and this higher dose is necessary to have an anti-cancer effect.

Case reports have been published since then which showed benefits from intravenous vitamin C against cancer. (53)

At a certain concentration, vitamin C stops acting like an antioxidant in the body and begins behaving like a pro-oxidant. In the pro-oxidant form, vitamin C gets inside cancer cells and turns into hydrogen peroxide. The hydrogen peroxide is capable of killing cancer cells, since they do not have the mechanism to withstand it. (54) As an added bonus, vitamin C is not thought to be harmful to healthy cells. This means that vitamin C is a powerful tool with a lot of potential upside but no real downside as far as we can tell.

Yet another benefit of high dose vitamin C is that it can make chemotherapy more effective in killing cancer cells. One notable study found that vitamin C potentiated the effect of several of the most commonly used drugs in breast cancer treatment. (55) In order to take advantage of this effect, I like to give high dose vitamin C on days before and/or after chemotherapy treatment to hopefully maximize its efficacy.

The data thus far on IV vitamin C is very encouraging. Out of the many natural therapies in integrative oncology's tool chest, intravenous vitamin C is perhaps the one that the conventional community is closest to embracing. However, as is the case with many alternative therapies, we need more research to better understand it. (56) Additional studies are needed to validate the positive effects we have seen in smaller studies and in clinical practice.

Pulsed Electromagnetic Field Therapy (PEMF)

We frequently talk about the metabolic component to our cells in terms of the glucose they use and the ATP they produce, but there is an electromagnetic component to our cells as well.

Our whole body, in fact, emits its own electromagnetic field. Each individual cell in our body has its own frequency, or resonance, that it needs in order to function properly. There is a theory that posits when a cell's resonance is thrown off as result of the myriad of electromagnetic exposures, such as cell phones, WiFi signals, microwaves, or computers, or via toxic exposures in our environment (i.e., chemicals in our food, water, air, etc.), or even emotional stressors, it can trigger abnormal cellular behavior. If this abnormal cellular behavior is allowed to persist, cancer develops. Cancer cells have been shown to have an abnormal resonance that differs from normal, healthy cells. Research in the 1930s by Dr. Harold Saxon Burr, an anatomy professor at the Yale University School of Medicine, found that tumors have different electrical properties than normal tissue, and that the appearance of cancer in mice occurred after a measurable change in the organism's electromagnetic field. (57) This supports the metabolic theory of cancer, and how cancer develops as a result of abnormal stressors at the cellular level.

Jerry Tennant, MD, a prominent researcher in the field of electromagnetics and health, states that human cells are designed to function at approximately -20 millivolts (mV). Interestingly, this corresponds to a pH of 7.35, which we know is within the body's narrow pH range. As this voltage decreases, as a result of various insults to cells, the cell's physiology changes for the worse. (58) When a cell does not function properly, it is not able to take in nutrients nor is it able to eliminate wastes. Continued unchecked, these cells are at significantly increased risk of becoming cancerous.

Pulsed Electromagnetic Field Therapy, abbreviated PEMF, is a very simple, painless, and non-invasive way to address abnormal resonance in cells. The procedure involves simply lying down on a therapy pad that is plugged into a piece of equipment that generates steady, rhythmic pulses that the patient barely feels. The strength and frequency of the pulses can be adjusted, depending on the patient's specific diagnosis. The intent is to bring any abnormal cellular resonance back into balance.

Another benefit of PEMF is that it has been shown to assist in making cell membranes more permeable. Often, we administer oxygen while the patients are receiving PEMF therapy with the intent of ushering more oxygen into the cells.

PEMF might sound like something out of a science fiction movie, but there is actually a good deal of science behind it. In fact, PEMF has a number indications, including uses for inflammation, chronic pain, and Lyme disease. This is a lesser-known therapy, but it has become an important addition to virtually all of my cancer treatment protocols. I have observed improved outcomes since adding this to our list of therapies, and research backs this up. An excellent summary of the research by Vadala et al reviewed the evidence for PEMF's effectiveness both in vitro and in vivo. (59) The study authors went on to note that PEMF is safe and non-invasive, as well as being non-toxic to healthy cells.

While studies on human cancer cells, as well as in animals with cancer, have been encouraging, studies in human patients have been limited. However, we do have some smaller studies which found PEMF to be beneficial for a variety of cancer types. (60, 61)

As with other alternative cancer therapies we have discussed, we have a therapy which has scientific backing for its effectiveness, which selectively harms cancer cells and not healthy cells, and does not seem to cause any notable side effects. Why wouldn't we use it?!? Unfortunately, it does not have the level of proof needed for the insurance coverage to incorporate it into conventional cancer treatment programs.

Oxidative Therapy

Along with a long list of other important discoveries about cancer and how it works, Otto Warburg discovered that cancer does not thrive in oxygen-rich environments; cancer prefers a low oxygen environment. This is known as hypoxia. In contrast, the body's healthy cells thrive with an abundance of oxygen. Research since Dr. Warburg's time has uncovered the profound role that hypoxia plays in the development of cancer, as well as its continued growth and metastasis. We now know that frequent and sustained hypoxia makes cancer cells more aggressive, and also regulates the environment around tumors to support cancer's growth and progression. (62)

When tumors do not have enough oxygen, and have used up all available oxygen, they are able to up-regulate the production of substances which promote angiogenesis. These new blood vessels which are formed serve to deliver additional oxygen to the tumor, as well as other growth factors. (63) To further complicate matters, it turns out that most all tumors have some areas of hypoxia and some areas of adequate oxygen supply. As a result, a combination of angiogenesis and oxidative stress exist, a phenomenon known as cycling hypoxia. Left unchecked, this influences response to treatment as well as metastatic behavior. (64)

Therapies designed to increase oxygen are collectively known as oxidative therapies. On the most basic level, deep breathing can be considered an oxidative therapy because extra oxygen is brought into the lungs and transported into the blood. We can all benefit from being more intentional about our breathing. However, for cancer fighting purposes, deep breathing alone is not likely going to be enough.

A step-up from simply breathing more deeply is to provide oxygen supplementally. This is given through the nose, using a nasal cannula. The cannula is a clear tube which connects to an oxygen tank. Although we typically think of this form of oxygen as being reserved for those with lung issues such as emphysema, I feel that it has a role in cancer treatment for most everyone. In my practice, I have patients on supplemental oxygen via nasal cannula when receiving certain therapies where we believe extra oxygen will improve efficacy. As mentioned earlier, PEMF is one such therapy.

A more substantial oxidative therapy is hyperbaric oxygen. Often abbreviated HBOT, hyperbaric oxygen therapy entails the administration of 100% oxygen at pressures which are higher than what is normally found in our earthly atmosphere. By giving 100% oxygen at pressures higher than normal, extra oxygen is delivered to the tissues and cells of the body. In order to achieve these higher atmospheric pressures, a hyperbaric chamber must be used.

Hyperbaric oxygen is routinely used in conventional medicine to accelerate wound healing, but it can be used as an off-label cancer treatment. Some scientists have expressed concern that additional oxygen could stimulate growth of cancer, rather than the inhibition of it. A thorough review of the existing literature found that hyperbaric oxygen does not promote cancer growth and proliferation. Additionally, HBOT was found to inhibit cancer growth in certain cancers. However, some cancer types, including cervical and bladder, seem to be non-responders to HBOT in studies thus far. (65)

While there is no one-size-fits-all treatment for cancer, I feel that hyperbaric oxygen can be a powerful component of many integrative cancer treatment protocols.

Photodynamic Therapy

Photodynamic therapy is a non-invasive treatment consisting of the administration of specific wavelengths of light in order to kill cancer cells. More specifically, photodynamic therapy uses infrared light in the 700 nm to 1 mm range. It is part of the electromagnetic spectrum, which includes both visible and invisible light. Infrared light is invisible to the human eye. It can, however, be felt as heat. Infrared light has the unique ability to penetrate the skin.

The key to photodynamic therapy lies in a photosensitizing agent which is strategically ingested prior to treatment and is taken up by cancer cells. This agent, which is non-toxic, primes the cancer cells so that they are susceptible to a photochemical reaction when exposed to a specific wavelength of light. The result is the death of cancer cells, leaving healthy cells unharmed.

Research has shown that photodynamic therapy is compatible with other treatments. Chemotherapy has been shown to improve the effectiveness of photodynamic therapy. (66) Celecoxib seems to potentiate the anti-tumor effects of photodynamic therapy. (67) Even vitamin D has been shown to enhance the effectiveness of photodynamic therapy. (68)

Because oxygen plays a vital role in the photodynamic therapy process, would it not make sense to combine it in the same treatment protocol with hyperbaric oxygen? Early research suggests that it could be a quite efficacious combination. (69) Clinical experience thus far tells us that photodynamic therapy is a very safe and effective therapy, which is compatible with other therapies as part of an integrative cancer treatment program.

Lymphatic Therapy

The lymphatic system has been largely forgotten about in conventional medicine, but it serves some very important purposes within the body. Namely, the lymphatic system serves as the training ground for our immune system. The lymphatic system runs in parallel to the blood stream, and when the bone marrow makes white blood cells, these new cells are ushered into the lymphatic system. Once in the lymphatic system, white blood cells learn how to protect the body against foreign pathogens. When those cells are properly trained, they are moved into the blood stream so that they can help the body fight foreign invaders.

With cancer patients, there is frequently some level of lymphatic dysfunction. This is certainly true in cancers which have spread to the lymph nodes. The surgical removal of lymph nodes is sure to result in congestion within the lymphatic system, reducing the flow of lymph and thus impairing the immune system. The extreme example of this is when we see a large swelling in an area, known as a lymphedema. Areas with the highest concentration of lymph nodes are the neck, the armpit, and the groin, but lymph nodes exist throughout the body. Lymphatic therapy is intended to break up the congested fluid, allowing for proper flow of lymph.

Lymphatic therapy can occur via multiple methods. Jumping on a rebounder or using a skin brush is an easy way to enhance lymph flow at home. More in-depth treatment can be achieved through a massage therapist trained in lymphatics.

The term, "lymphatic drainage," was first coined by Dr. Frederic Millard, a physician from Canada, in the 1920s. (70) By the 1930s, a husband and wife team, Drs. Emil and Estrid Vodder, developed lymph drainage therapy further. (71) That method was subsequently perfected by a French physician named Dr. Bruno Chikly, and is the basis for the form of lymph drainage we use today. (72) Dr. Chikly notes that lymph drainage therapy provides several crucial benefits, including: stimulation of the immune system; elimination of toxins; enhancement of the nervous system; and improved circulation of various fluids, including lymph, interstitial fluid, cerebrospinal fluid, and blood.

I have personally witnessed some incredible results in my patients as a result of lymph drainage therapy. Some patients have come into the office, not being able to lift their arms above horizontal level due to lymphedema. After only a couple weeks of bi-weekly treatment, much of their mobility problems were rectified by using lymph drainage therapy. In addition to improved range of motion in lymphedema, I also believe that lymph drainage plays a key role in helping the body fight cancer and detoxify. As an added bonus, a lymphatic drainage session is also very calming and relaxing.

•————————————•

(1)   Skipper HE, Schabel FM, Mellett LB, et al. Implications of biochemical, cytokinetic, pharmacologic, and toxicologic relationships in the design of optimal therapeutic schedules. Cancer Chemother Rep 1970; 54: 431-50.

(2)   Fidler IJ, Ellis LM. Chemotherapeutic drugs - more really is not better. Nat Med 2000; 6(5): 500-2.

(3)   Hanahan D, Bergers G, Bergsland E. Less is more, regularly: metronomic dosing of cytotoxic drugs can target tumor angiogenesis in mice. J Clin Invest 2000; 105: 1045-7.

(4) Kareva I, Waxman DJ, Klement GL. Metronomic chemotherapy: an attractive alternative to maximum tolerated dose therapy that can activate anti-tumor immunity and minimize therapeutic resistance. Cancer Lett 2015; 358(2): 100-6.

(5) Browder T, Butterfield CE, Kraling BM, et al. Antiangiogenic scheduling of chemotherapy improves efficacy against experimental drug-resistant cancer. Cancer Res 2000; 60(7): 1878-86.

(6) Klement G, Baruchel S, Ran J, et al. Continuous low-dose therapy with vinblastine and VEGF receptor-2 antibody induces sustained tumor regression without overt toxicity. J Clin Invest 2000; 105(8): R15-24.

(7) Ayre SG, Garcia y Bellon DP, Garcia DP Jr. Insulin, chemotherapy, and the mechanisms of malignancy: the design and demise of cancer. Med Hypotheses 2000; 55(4): 330-34.

(8) Holmes MD, Chen WY. Hiding in plain view: the potential for commonly used drugs to reduce breast cancer mortality. Breast Cancer Res 2012; 14(6): 216.

(9) Libby G, Donnelly LA, Donnan PT, et al. New users of Metformin are at low risk of incident cancer: a cohort study among people with type 2 diabetes. Diabetes Care 2009; 32(9): 1620-5.

(10) Chiang GG, Abraham RT. Targeting the mTOR signaling network in cancer. Trends Mol Med 2007; 13: 433-42.

(11) Guertin DA, Sabatini DM. Defining the role of mTOR in cancer. Cancer Cell 2007 Jul; 12(1): 9-22.

(12) LeRoith D, Roberts CT. Insulin-like growth factors and cancer. Ann Intern Med 1995; 122: 54-9.

(13) Redman BG, Esper P, Pan Q, et al. Phase II trial of tetrathiomolybdate in patients with advanced kidney cancer. Clin Cancer Res 2003; 9(5): 1666-72.

(14) Wang JS and Groopman J. DNA damage by mycotoxins. Mutation Research 1999; 424: 167-81.

(15) Liu Y and Wu F. Global burden of aflatoxin-induced hepatocellular carcinoma: a risk assessment. Environmental Health Perspectives 2010; 118: 818-24.

(16) Antonarakis ES, Heath EL, Smith DC, et al. Repurposing itraconazole as a treatment for advanced prostate cancer: a noncooperative randomized phase II trial in men with metastatic castration-resistant prostate cancer. Oncologist 2013; 18(2): 163-73.

(17) Holmes NE, Charles PGP. Safety and Efficacy Review of Doxycycline. Clin Med Insights Ther 2009; 1: 471-82.

(18) De Francesco EM, Bonuccelli G, Maggiolini M, et al. Vitamin C and doxycycline: a synthetic lethal combination therapy targeting metabolic flexibility in cancer stem cells (CSCs). Oncotarget 2017; 8(40): 67269-86.

(19) Lamb R, Fiorillo M, Chadwick A, et al. Doxycycline down-regulates DNA-PK and radiosensitizes tumor initiating cells: Implications for more effective radiation therapy. Oncotarget 2015; 6(16): 14005-25.

(20) Adams WJ, Morris DL. Short-course cimetidine and survival with colorectal cancer. Lancet 1994; 344: 8939-8940.

(21) Nagano T, Matsuda H, Park YC, et al. Successful treatment of metastatic renal cell carcinoma with cimetidine - report of two cases. Nihon Hinyokika Gakkai Zasshi 1996;87(10):1201-4.

(22) Borgstrom S, et al. Human leukocyte interferon and cimetidine for metastatic melanoma. N Engl J Med 1982; 307(17): 1080-1081.

(23) Katoh J, et al. Cimetidine reduces impairment of cellular immunity after cardiac operations with cardiopulmonary bypass. J Thorac Cardiovasc Surg 1998; 116(2): 312-318.

(24) Dumont FJ, Su Q. Mechanism of action of the immunosuppressant rapamycin. Life Sci 1996; 58(5): 373-95.

(25) Cohen EEW, Wu K, Hartford C, et al. Phase 1 studies of sirolimus alone or in combination with pharmacokinetic modulators in advanced cancer patients. Clin Cancer Res 2012; 18(17): 4785-93.

(26) Law BK. Rapamycin: an anti-cancer immunosuppressant? Crit Rev Oncol Hematol 2005; 56(1): 47-60.

(27) Ke Y, Ye K, Grossniklaus HE, et al. Noscapine inhibits tumor growth with little toxicity to normal tissues or inhibition of immune responses. Cancer Immunol Immunother 2000; 49(4-5): 217-25.

(28) Newcomb EW, Lukyanov Y, Schnee T, et al. Noscapine inhibits hypoxia-mediated HIF-1alpha expression and angiogenesis in vitro: a novel function for an old drug. Int J Oncol 2006; 28(5): 1121-30.

(29) Sauna ZE, Shukla S, and Ambudkar SV. Disulfiram, an old drug with new potential therapeutic uses for human cancers and fungal infections. Mol BioSyst 2005; 1: 127-34.

(30) Todd KE, Gloor B, Lane JS, et al. Resection of locally advanced pancreatic cancer after down staging with continuous-infusion 5-fluoruracil, mitomycin-C, leucovorin, and dipyridamole. J Gastrointest Surg 1998; 2(2): 159-66.

(31) Yatsunami J, Fukuno Y, Nagata M, et al. Anti-angiogenic and anti-tumor effects of 14-membered ring macrolides on mouse B16 melanoma cells. Clin Exp Metastasis 1999; 17(4): 361-7.

(32) Mikasa K, Sawaki M, Kita E, et al. Significant survival benefit to patients with advanced non-small-cell lung cancer from treatment with clarithromycin. Chemotherapy 1997; 43(4): 288-96.

(33) Mathews PM, Froelich CJ, Sibbitt WL, et al. Enhancement of natural cytotoxicity by beta-endorphin. J Immune 1983; 130(4): 1658-62.

(34) Garcia-Albeniz X, Chan AT. Aspirin for the prevention of colorectal cancer. Best Practices Res Clin Gastroenterol 2011; 25(0): 461-72.

(35)   Elwood PC, Morgan G, Pickering JE, et al. Aspirin in the treatment of cancer: reductions in metastatic spread and in mortality: a systematic review and meta-analyses of published studies. PLoS One 2016; 11(4): e0152402.

(36)   Perron L, Bairati I, Harel F, et al. Antihypertensive drug use and the risk of prostate cancer (Canada). Cancer Causes Control 2004; 15(6): 535-41.

(37)   Zhong S, Yu D, Zhang X, et al. B-Blocker use and morality in cancer patients: systematic review and meta-analysis of observational studies. Eur J Cancer Prev 2016; 25(5): 440-8.

(38)   Sloan EK, Priceman SJ, Cox BF, et al. The sympathetic nervous system induces a metastatic switch in primary breast cancer. Cancer Res 2010; 70(18): 7042-52.

(39)   Poynter JN, Gruber SB, Higgins PDR, et al. Statins and the risk of colorectal cancer. N Engl J Med 2005; 352: 2184-92.

(40)   Khurana V, Bejjanki HR, Caldito G, et al. Statins reduce the risk of lung cancer in humans: a large case-control study of US veterans. Chest 2007; 131(5): 1282-8.

(41)   Bansal D, Undela K, D'Cruz S, et al. Statin use and risk of prostate cancer: a meta-analysis of observational studies. PLoS One 2012; 7(10): e46691.

(42)   Kawata S, Yamasaki E, Nagase T, et al. Effect of pravastatin on survival in patients with advanced hepatocellular carcinoma. A randomized clinical trial. Br J Cancer 2001; 84(7): 886-91.

(43)   Hamilton RJ, Banez LL, Aronson WJ, et al. Statin medication use and the risk of biochemical recurrence after radical prostatectomy. Cancer 2010; 116(14): 3389-98.

(44)   Rofstad EK, Mathiesen B, et al. Acidic extracellular pH promotes experimental metastasis of human melanoma cells in athymic nude mice. Cancer Res 2006; 66(13): 6699-6707.

(45) Pilon-Thomas S, Kodumudi K, et al. Neutralization of Tumor Acidity Improves Antitumor Responses to Immunotherapy. Cancer Res 2015; 76(6): 1381-90.

(46) Sagiv E, Sheffer M, Shapira S, et al. Pathways of inflammation and carcinogenesis are activated in tumors but not normal tissues. Digestion 2011; 84: 169-84.

(47) Yu L, Wu WK, Li ZJ, et al. Enhancement of doxorubicin cytotoxicity on human esophageal squamous cell carcinoma cells by indomethacin and 4-[5-(4-chlorophenyl)-3-(trifluoromethyl)-1H-pyrazol-1-yl]benzenesulfonamide (SC236) via inhibiting P-glycoprotein activity. Mol Pharmacol 2009; 75(6): 1364-73.

(48) Lev-Ari S, Strier L, Kazanov D, et al. Celecoxib and curcumin synergistically inhibit the growth of colorectal cancer cells. Clin Cancer Res 2005; 11(18): 6738-44.

(49) Hardtner C, Multhoff G, Falk W, et al. Epigallocatechin-3-gallate, a green tea-derived catechin, synergizes with celecoxib to inhibit IL-1-induced tumorigenic mediators by human pancreatic adenocarcinoma cells Colo357. Eur J Pharmacy 2012; 684(1-3): 36-43.

(50) Putchala MC, Ramani P, Premukmar P, et al. Ascorbic acid and its pro-oxidant activity as a therapy for tumours of oral cavity - a systematic review. Arch Oral Biol 213; 58(6): 563-74.

(51) Cameron E, Campbell A. The orthomolecular treatment of cancer. II. Clinical trial of high-dose ascorbic acid supplements in advanced human cancer. Chem Biol Interact 1974; 9(4): 285-315.

(52) Mortal CG, Fleming TR, Creagan ET, et al. High-dose vitamin C versus placebo in the treatment of patients with advanced cancer who have had no prior chemotherapy. A randomized double-blind comparison. N Engl J Med 1985; 312(3): 137-41.

(53) Padayatty SJ, Riordan HD, Hewitt SM, et al. Intravenously administered vitamin C as cancer therapy: three cases. Canadian Medical Association Journal 2006; 174(7): 937-42.

(54) Du J, Cullen JJ, Buettner GR. Ascorbic acid: chemistry, biology, and the treatment of cancer. Biochim Biophys Acta 2012; 1826(2): 443-57.

(55) Kurbacher CM, Wagner U, Kolster B, Andreotti PE, Krebs D, Bruckner HW: Ascorbic Acid (Vitamin C) improves the Antineoplastic Activity of Doxorubicin, Cisplatin, and Paclitaxel in Human Breast Carcinoma Cells in Vitro. Cancer Letters 1996; 103: 183-9.

(56) Fritz H, Flower G, Weeks L, et al. Intravenous Vitamin C and Cancer: A Systematic Review. Integr Cancer Ther 2014; 13(4): 280-300.

(57) Burr HS, Smith GM, Strong LC. Bioelectric properties of cancer-resistant and cancer-susceptible mice. Am J Cancer 1938; 32: 240-48.

(58) Tennant J. Healing is Voltage: Cancer's On/Off Switches: Polarity. CreateSpace, 2015. Print.

(59) Vadala M, Morales-Medina JC, Vallelunga A, et al. Mechanisms and therapeutic effectiveness of pulsed electromagnetic field therapy in oncology. Cancer Med 2016; 5(11): 3128-39.

(60) Barbault A, Costa FP, Bottger B, et al. Amplitude-modulated electromagnetic fields for the treatment of cancer: discovery of tumor-specific frequencies and assessment of a novel therapeutic approach. J Exp Clin Cancer Res 2009; 28: 51.

(61) Costa FP, de Oliviera AC, Meirelles R, et al. Treatment of advanced hepatocellular carcinoma with very low levels of amplitude-modulated electromagnetic fields. Br J Cancer 2011; 105: 640-8.

(62) Muz B, de la Puente P, Azab F, et al. The role of hypoxia in cancer progression, angiogenesis, metastasis, and resistance to therapy. Hypoxia (Auckl) 2015; 3: 83-92.

(63) Sermenza GL. Hypoxia-inducible factors: mediators of cancer progression and targets for cancer therapy. Trends Pharmacy Sci 2012; 33: 207-14.

(64) Dewhirst MW. Relationships between cycling hypoxia, HIF-1, angiogenesis and oxidative stress. Radiat Res 2009; 172(6): 653-65.

(65) Moen I, Stuhr LE. Hyperbaric oxygen therapy and cancer - a review. Target Oncol 2012; 7(4): 233-42.

(66) Nahabedian MY, Cohen RA, Contino MF, et al. Combination cytotoxic chemotherapy with cisplatin or doxorubicin and photodynamic therapy in murine tumors. J Nat Cancer Inst 1988; 80: 739-43.

(67) Ferrario A, Fisher AM, Rucker N, et al. Celecoxib and NS-398 enhance photodynamic therapy by increasing in vitro apoptosis and decreasing in vivo inflammatory and angiogenic factors. Cancer Res 2005; 65: 9473-8.

(68) Sato N, Moore BW, Keevey S, et al. Vitamin D enhances ALA-induced protoporphyrin IX production and photodynamic cell death in 3-D organotypic cultures of keratinocytes. J Invest Dermatol 2007; 127: 925-34.

(69) Matzi VMA, Sankin O, Lindenmann J, et al. Photodynamic therapy enhanced by hyperbaric oxygenation in palliation of malignant pleural mesothelioma: clinical experience. Photodiagnosis and Photodynamic Therapy 2004: 57-64.

(70) Millard FP. Applied Anatomy of the Lymphatics. Kirksville: International Lymphatic Research Society, 1922.French, Ramona Moody. The Complete Guide to Lymph Drainage Massage, Clifton Park: Milady, 2011.

(71) French, RM. The Complete Guide to Lymph Drainage Massage, Clifton Park: Milady, 2011.

(72) Chikly, Bruno. Lymph Drainage Therapy and its integration in a massage therapy practice. American Massage Therapy Association, page 20. URL http://www.iahe.com/images/pdf/3319_001.pdf.

CHAPTER 6

The Role of Nutrition in Cancer Prevention and Treatment

"Let food be thy medicine, and medicine be thy food."
— Hippocrates

You Are What You Eat

One of the myths perpetuated by conventional oncology—and one I sincerely hope that this book can assist in dispelling—is that cancer is largely a disease of genetics. This myth would have us believe that regardless of other factors, or any preventative measures a person takes, if you "have cancer in your family" or are unlucky enough to inherit faulty DNA from mom or dad, you are doomed to receive a cancer diagnosis. Realistically, we can only say with certainty that about 6-8% of cancers are purely genetic in origin. (1) This leaves us with an overwhelming majority of cancers with an underlying cause that is not the result of genetics. Simply put, environmental factors, or what we expose ourselves to on a daily basis, play a critical role in our risk for developing cancer. We can thus extrapolate that the foods we consume are a big portion of our environment.

It has long been known that diet plays a role in diseases like heart disease and diabetes, and that knowledge has woven its way into the advice on prevention given by cardiologists and endocrinologists for some time now. However, as we have discussed, there is shockingly little advice offered by oncologists when it comes to nutrition as a tool for cancer prevention. This is frustrating, particularly in light of the fact that it is estimated that between 40-50% of cancer cases could be prevented with some simple lifestyle changes. Dietary changes are a significant portion of these controllable lifestyle factors. (2)

Similarly, there is little by way of dietary advice from conventional oncology when it comes to nutrition as a tool in cancer treatment. Most oncologists offer no advice, and many wrongfully claim that it really does not matter what you eat, so long as you do not lose too much weight. We do know, however, from a number of studies, that nutrition can play a role in improved outcomes. People who eat better do better in terms treatment and mitigation of side effects from treatment. (3)

On the other side of this debate, there is a good deal of misinformation about the role of diet in both cancer prevention and cancer treatment. The internet is full of anecdotes of people curing their cancer using diet alone. Much of this information likely exists somewhere between being extreme exaggeration or flat-out misinformation. Ultimately, much of the published literature confirms that using diet as a sole means of cancer treatment is largely ineffective. (4) This has not stopped the internet from being littered with unconfirmed accounts of miraculous healing using diet alone to fight cancer. I am personally aware of people who have beaten cancer with nutrition alone, but these represent a very small minority of patients. In contrast, I know many, many more individuals who have attempted to treat cancer with nutrition alone and have failed. Is it possible to defeat cancer with nutrition alone? Absolutely—but it is not likely.

In integrative oncology, we take a pragmatic and science-based approach to using nutrition in our treatment protocols. It is beneficial to think of the body as a garden. Some of the more powerful treatment tools, such as surgery, chemotherapy, and radiation are beneficial at removing the cancerous "weeds" from the body. Diet, however, is a way of making the soil less hospitable to those weeds, making them less likely to grow and flourish. Those weeds likely would not have grown, however, if the terrain inside the body was not hospitable to their growth to begin with. This is where diet becomes a powerful tool for cancer prevention. The role of diet in cancer prevention is to alter the terrain, making it difficult for cancer to form or flourish.

One of the empowering aspects of nutrition is that it is definitely in our control. Accepting the fact that dietary habits likely played a role in getting cancer is often a tough pill to swallow. However, with that knowledge comes the realization that nutritional choices can also play a powerful role in cancer treatment. One of the greatest fears many patients have about cancer treatment is that they are limited in what they can do themselves. Nutrition provides a directly controllable factor for patients, allowing them to play an integral part in their own treatment, and thus potentially affecting the outcome in a positive way.

Do You Know What Is in Your Food?

This is a profoundly important question we should all be asking ourselves. What we eat is such an important part of our life and health, but often, we do not think twice about what, or how much, we put into our mouths. Most of us in the developed world have grown up with an abundance of food throughout all seasons, often at arm's length, and this has led to a level of complacency—and quite frankly, ignorance—about what is actually in the food we eat. Likely, if we knew what was in some of the food we ate on a daily basis and what the subsequent health implications are for consuming such food regularly, our diets would likely look dramatically different. It is time to develop mindfulness about what we all eat.

There are over 2,500 chemical additives that are used in food, and an additional 12,000 chemical substances have the possibility of finding their way into our food, whether through environmental contamination or as a result of producing food. (5) According to Dr. Larry McCleary, a physician, researcher, and author, "About eighty percent of the food on the shelves of supermarkets today didn't exist 100 years ago." (6) This is a staggering statistic regarding the reality in which we now live; where food is rarely healthy fuel for our bodies, but instead, artificial, chemically-laden poison. Simply reading the ingredients list on the back of the label of many of the processed foods people eat every day reveals a long list of ingredients with difficult-to-pronounce names. Often, these ingredients are preservatives, stabilizers, or other non-food ingredients used to preserve color or shelf life. Many of these are ingredients we should strive to avoid, as they are not even technically food themselves.

Food Additives to Avoid

With so many food additives, it is impossible to list them all, or have a comprehensive assessment of each food additive's carcinogenicity here. Truly, even the industries that use or manufacture these chemicals, and the researchers tasked with determining their safety, likely do not fully understand the risks associated with the use of these chemicals over the long-term. Often, it seems like we are the guinea pigs. The best course of action is likely to avoid food additives, altogether, when possible. While this list is by no means comprehensive, there are some food additives I can confidently recommend avoiding completely. When possible, it is best to avoid any and all food additives that are not food, themselves.

BHA and BHT

Both butylated hydroxyanisole (BHA) and butylated hydroxytoluene (BHT) are similar but individual preservatives often used in combination with one another. BHA is considered "reasonably anticipated to be carcinogenic to humans," yet it is still considered GRAS (generally recognized as safe) by the FDA. BHT has been reported to trigger certain cancers in rats, but human studies are lacking. Both are considered to likely be endocrine disruptors. (7)

Propyl Paraben

Propyl paraben is added to foods like muffins and tortillas. It has been shown to be an endocrine disruptor and can influence genes important in breast cancers, and accelerate those cancer cells' growth. (7)

Sodium Nitrite

In the early part of the 20th century, gastric cancers were among the most prevalent cancers and were the leading cause of cancer-related deaths. During that time, curing meat with high amounts of sodium—including sodium nitrite—was the most common method of preservation. Ultimately, it was concluded that the high levels of sodium nitrite played a key role in the high rates of gastric cancers.

Despite the fact that we know sodium nitrite can play a role in gastric cancers, it is still commonly used in many kinds of cured and processed meats, such as bacon, lunch meats, hot dogs, and sausages.

Chemical Contaminants

Often, what contaminates our food is likely more worrisome than the listed ingredients. Toxic contaminants such as mercury, cadmium, other heavy metals, and industrial pollutants can infiltrate certain foods, especially fish. Hormones and antibiotics often contaminate other kinds of animal products, such as dairy and meats. Even the containers in which foods are sold and stored, such as plastic bottles and aluminum cans, can leach chemicals into our food. Pesticides used in conventional produce have also been shown to be potentially carcinogenic, and ultimately find their way to our dinner plates.

As with food additives, it is impossible to list all the chemicals that can inadvertently wind up in our food. The best course of action is to be aware of the risk of certain contaminants, and mitigate that risk as best as we can. The below list is by no means comprehensive, but represents a small number of the chemical contaminants found in foods that likely influence cancer risk.

Aflatoxins

Aflatoxins are among the most carcinogenic, naturally-occurring substances. Aflatoxins are secondary metabolites of certain fungi and molds that can infest certain kinds of foods, including corn, peanuts, cottonseed (and cottonseed oil). Aflatoxins can also contaminate dairy products, eggs, nuts, almonds, and certain spices. Aflatoxins are known to cause liver cancer in humans, among a variety of other health problems. (8)

BPA

BPA, or bisphenol A, is a component used to make the polycarbonate and plastic packaging used for many kinds of food, but it is also present in plasticware, plastic cups and other plastics used in the kitchen. It is in the plastics that are commonly used to line aluminum cans. Bisphenol A can leach into food when plastic becomes too hot, too cold, gets scratched, or otherwise damaged. Many regulatory agencies, such as the FDA, tell us that the levels of BPA found in food are likely not harmful (9), but other research suggests that BPA can play a role in cancer development. (10) BPA acts as an endocrine disruptor; endocrine disruptors are thought to influence certain hormone-dependent cancers, such as prostate and breast cancer.

Glyphosate (Roundup)

Glyphosate, or Roundup, is among the most heavily used pesticides in all of history. Manufactured by Monsanto, for years we were told by the company that glyphosate was safe and that their own internal research confirmed its safety and efficacy. We now know that glyphosate is carcinogenic. (11) The risk of cancer is higher for farm workers regularly exposed to glyphosate, but this does not mean we should be complacent about glyphosate—or any other pesticides—in our food. A little bit of exposure over the course of many years is likely still something to be concerned about.

rBGH

Recombinant bovine growth hormone (rBGH) is also known as recombinant bovine somatotropin (rBST), and is a synthetic form of bovine growth hormone given to dairy cows to increase milk production. Subsequently, the dairy products from cows treated with these hormones are tainted with these hormones, including insulin-like growth factor 1 (IGF-1), a hormone known to play a role in hormone dependent cancers. (12) These hormones have been banned in Europe, Canada, and other parts of the world, but the United States continues to allow their use.

Unsurprisingly, industry and even some of our own regulatory agencies downplay the potential harm of these additives and contaminants, as their goal is to maximize production and prolong the shelf life of their products as much as possible. But we must ask ourselves: do we really know what the cumulative effect is of all of these contaminants in our food? We know for certain that certain unnatural ingredients and many environmental pollutants are harmful to our health, but could all of these things really lead to cancer?

It is important to remember that the cumulative effect of all of these environmental factors is what we are concerned about when it comes to eating a diet that protects against cancer. Our cells can only withstand so many "hits" until our toxic bucket overflows, making the development of cancer more likely.

Needless to say, the quality of our food is extremely important. Where our food comes from, how it is produced, and how it is stored are all important factors to consider when trying to eat in a way that protects against cancer. Assuming that our food is safe, simply because it ends up in a grocery store or a restaurant, is a dangerous approach to take when it comes to health.

Knowing what is in the food that you prepare and eat at home is one thing, but knowing what you are getting when you go out to eat is quite another. Eating out regularly—even the majority of the time—has become commonplace for many people, which is a relatively new phenomenon. It is much harder to guarantee that the food you are getting is of high quality when you eat out; you simply cannot always know what is in your food. Restaurants' goal is to run a business; while they have a vested interest in making their food delicious, it is not always the goal to have the highest quality of ingredients, or to ensure that the food they serve is healthy.

If we are going to eat in a way that works to prevent cancer, it is important to know where our food comes from, and what is in it. Eating out must become more of an occasional occurrence, rather than a regular practice. For those who are actively fighting cancer, purchasing the highest quality food yourselves and preparing food at home should be the rule, with very few exceptions.

Tips on How to Avoid Food Additives and Dangerous Chemical Contaminants

- Avoid processed foods. These foods are where you will most likely find the wide variety of food additives.
- Avoid cured meats, including bacon, ham, lunch meats, and sausage.
- Eat organic whenever possible. You will be avoiding many of the harmful pesticides inherent in conventionally grown foods.
- Be mindful about how and where the food you buy was sourced.
- Avoid foods commonly contaminated with mycotoxins, such as corn, wheat and peanuts.

How Now Shall We Eat?

Nutrition, particularly with regard to cancer, can be a difficult issue to address because there is so much information available. Frustratingly, much of the information is conflicting. Given nutrition's importance, it's something we must address. The necessary task of sifting through nutritional data underscores the importance of the integrative oncologist's experience and training in cancer treatment, and how nutrition can influence treatment.

It is important to note that a cancer prevention diet and a diet that is used in cancer treatment are very similar. Therefore, this information becomes a valuable tool not just for cancer patients, but also for anyone who seeks to prevent cancer. In the case of cancer treatment, patients are expected to maintain the strictest version of my anti-cancer diet. Remember, we are using diet as a means to support the internal terrain of the body, making cancer development and proliferation more difficult. As mentioned previously, diet should be viewed as a powerful cancer treatment, which is supportive in nature rather than an exclusive treatment itself.

It is also important to note that our recommendations on diet should (and likely will) shift over time somewhat, as new research emerges. This is a healthy attitude, and unfortunately one that is not necessarily shared by many in conventional oncology, or mainstream medicine, for that matter.

Choosing a Diet and Common Sense

Much of the dietary advice I used to give patients centered around what is known as the ketogenic diet. The ketogenic diet focuses on macronutrient proportions; in other words, what is the percentage of fat, carbohydrates and protein in overall caloric intake? The ketogenic diet seeks to eliminate virtually all carbohydrates, comprising approximately 5% of total caloric intake. It allows for a moderate amount of protein (approximately 20% of total daily intake), with a focus on a high amount of fat (approximately 75% of total daily intake).

Naturally, the ketogenic diet focuses on foods high in fat, such as oils, avocados, nuts, seeds, and butter. Vegetables are encouraged on the ketogenic diet, but most fruits and vegetables high in carbohydrates or natural sugars (such as carrots, sweet potatoes, beets, etc.) are discouraged in the name of meeting the proper macronutrient proportions. Legumes, grains, and some dairy are excluded in the ketogenic diet as well, since they contain carbohydrates.

There has been a good deal of research done on the ketogenic diet with regard to weight loss, and for some people, the ketogenic diet is very effective toward this end. For cancer prevention, we know that maintaining a healthy weight is beneficial; in cancer treatment, however, we are not necessarily wanting patients to lose weight. Much of the thrust behind my recommendation for the ketogenic diet, however, centered around research that it might be beneficial in cancer treatment. There have been some promising studies done on the ketogenic diet's role in that regard. (13) Given what we know about cancer's metabolism and heavy reliance on sugar, it makes sense that the ketogenic diet might confer some of these anti-cancer benefits.

The ketogenic diet, however, is not without some problems. Many people find it difficult to conform to such a diet. Eating a very high fat diet, with only moderate protein and almost no carbohydrates, while also eating at a caloric deficit, can be extremely challenging. Since it is the responsibility of the patient to maintain the prescribed diet, this is a problem, and we must be pragmatic about the type of diet we recommend. The most effective diet in the world is ineffective if it is unable to be properly followed by a patient, so this must be taken into consideration.

More importantly, I am not convinced that the ketogenic diet is necessarily the best or most effective diet to use against cancer. Since the vast majority of daily calories must come from fat on the ketogenic diet, many people turn to foods like meats and cheeses to meet their daily calorie intake. Even if you add in some vegetables, this does not constitute a healthy diet, nor does it necessarily constitute a diet that is conducive to fighting cancer. Furthermore, many of the foods that are discouraged on the ketogenic diet are excellent sources of cancer-fighting nutrients and antioxidants, and it is inappropriate to exclude these in my opinion. These include certain fruits, vegetables, legumes, and some grains.

To that end, there has been a good deal of research indicating that plant-based diets confer numerous health benefits, particularly with regard to cancer. One of the most cited of these studies is detailed in a book entitled, The China Study. The book was written by T. Colin Campbell, a nutritional biochemist and professor at Cornell University, and his son, Thomas M. Campbell, a physician, and was based on an epidemiological study conducted in 65 counties in China. Ultimately, the authors concluded that people who ate a plant-based diet were less likely to die from cancer, among other "Western" diseases.

Are we to deduce that the benefits of a plant-based diet are due to the foods which are included, the foods which are excluded, or a combination of both? It is important to use our common sense when formulating a cancer fighting nutrition plan. What can we deduce from the research on these very different, specific diets in conjunction with what we know to be true about cancer? When we do this, we see commonalities and patterns develop.

Certainly, some of the benefit conferred from a diet such as the ketogenic diet comes from the elimination of high-glycemic foods. High glycemic foods are foods that are high in simple carbohydrates (rapidly absorbed glucose) that prompt a dramatic insulin response. Since we know that cancer cells have a much higher number of insulin and sugar receptors compared to normal cells, we can confidently say that eliminating high glycemic foods is likely an important strategy when fighting cancer.

Conversely, much of the anti-cancer benefit conferred by a plant-based diet is likely the result of the rich antioxidant and phytonutrient content inherent in such a diet. Even though some of these foods might be higher in carbohydrates, many of them are rich in fiber, which lessens their glycemic impact. This is an important distinction from high-glycemic foods, which are not buffered by fiber. Still, some foods in spite of their higher sugar and carbohydrate content (such as carrots, beets, and sweet potatoes), have shown benefit against cancer. Should we not include these kinds of foods in an anti-cancer diet?

It is my belief that naturally-occurring carbohydrates found in fruit, vegetables, and grains are processed and absorbed by the body differently than manmade sugars such as high fructose corn syrup. Although both categories are considered carbohydrates, they are almost certainly not created equal. We see the same thing with fats, where the naturally-occurring fats from coconuts, avocados, and olives are viewed much differently than man-made fats such as trans fats.

What Should We Restrict?

While the information surrounding nutrition's role in cancer can be conflicting, there are a wide variety of foods I can confidently recommend restricting (or at times, eliminating) as part of an anti-cancer diet.

Genetically Modified Foods

There is much hype over genetically modified organisms (GMOs), and controversy exists as to whether or not they are safe. Unfortunately, we do not have the benefit of long-term studies confirming or denying their health effects. What we do know, however, is that GMOs are often modified for the explicit purpose of being resistant to pesticides, which can then be dumped en masse on these crops. To that end, we know that pesticide products like glyphosate elevate cancer risk, and are something we should avoid. (11) Given that we do not have laws forcing food purveyors to label GMOs in the United States, the best way to avoid GMOs is to buy organic whenever possible. Any food labeled with the USDA Organic label cannot be genetically modified.

Some foods are more likely to be genetically modified than others, particularly soy, corn, rice, tomatoes, beets, potatoes, canola oil, papayas and yellow squash. (14) Some of these you should likely be avoiding because of their high glycemic index or heavy processing (canola oil), but in the case of foods such as tomatoes, it is best to opt for organic sources whenever possible.

Gluten

Gluten is the protein found in wheat. Many people are intolerant to gluten and do not even know it. For some, that intolerance is strong enough to be considered an allergy, which is what we see in Celiac disease. We have known for some time that people who are allergic to gluten who do not eliminate it from their diet are at a heightened risk for developing cancer. (15)

Many people tolerate gluten just fine, but there is evidence that it is mildly inflammatory even in those who do not have an allergy or intolerance to it. The fact is that much of the wheat and grain available to use today is far different from what our ancestors ate. Because almost all wheat commercially available has been hybridized from its original form, I typically recommend that cancer patients eliminate gluten-containing grains altogether. The only exception to this is sprouted grains, such as those found in Ezekiel 4:9 bread. For those without a gluten allergy or insensitivity, sprouted grains—though they do contain gluten—are acceptable since they provide some excellent health benefits. Sprouted grains, in contrast to non-sprouted grains, have higher fiber content, more absorbable vitamins and minerals, and are also easier to digest.

It is important to note that not all grains contain gluten; oats, quinoa, amaranth, and buckwheat do not contain gluten. These grains are acceptable, and in fact, encouraged.

One final point: most products marketed as "gluten free" are not healthy at all, despite being free of gluten. Read labels carefully!

High Glycemic Foods

It is essential to exclude high glycemic index foods. This includes high fructose corn syrup, sugar, evaporated cane juice, brown rice syrup, and any of the other names sugar hides behind. Cancer thrives on sugar, something that is particularly abundant in the Western diet. It is estimated that people in the United States consume over 75 pounds of sugar each year! (16) Many patients ask me if naturally-occurring high glycemic foods such as honey, maple syrup, and molasses are acceptable. I believe they are okay in moderation, but my preference is that they be minimized since they do cause a rapid rise in blood sugar (and thus insulin).

Many of the foods that people eat every day contain added sugar, often in high amounts. This includes sodas, sports drinks, juices, salad dressings, processed snack foods, and even many of the "healthy" granola bars, energy bars, and protein bars. Awareness of what is in your food becomes critical. Most people simply do not realize how much sugar they consume on a daily basis.

Other foods, such as refined carbohydrates, are at the top of the list of high glycemic foods. These include foods made with processed grains, including virtually all breads and pastas. Other carbohydrates, such as white rice and white potatoes, have a high glycemic index, and should ideally be minimized if not avoided completely.

Methionine

Methionine is an amino acid which is naturally present in many foods. Methionine is considered one of the eight essential amino acids, however it has the distinction of being the only essential amino acid in which its absence is still compatible with life. (17) This is because the body's healthy cells can produce methionine from other sources, including homocysteine. Thus, there is no known danger in restricting methionine in the diet.

More importantly, there is ample evidence that we should restrict methionine, especially as it relates to cancer treatment. Landmark research over 40 years ago found that normal cells in a Petri dish can grow just fine without methionine, but cancer cells cannot. (18) Studies since then have confirmed this finding that methionine restriction results in the death of cancer cells, but not normal cells. (19) This finding has also been seen in cancerous tumors, whereby tumors from a variety of different locations in the body were found to be dependent upon methionine for survival. (20)

There is not a drug or supplement to reduce or block methionine, so in order to minimize methionine levels in the body, we must reduce our consumption of methionine-containing foods. I feel strongly that restricting methionine is an essential anti-cancer nutritional strategy. Foods with the highest methionine content include fish, eggs, chicken, tuna, beef, pork, sesame seeds, cheese, and Brazil nuts. Foods with virtually no methionine include vegetables, fruits, and legumes. Armed with this knowledge, we have one more reason why plant-based diets are superior for fighting cancer.

There is no established cutoff for methionine when it comes to fighting cancer, nor is it practical or necessary to avoid methionine completely. However, eating high methionine foods on a limited basis, while emphasizing low methionine foods, is a no-brainer strategy based on the research I have read.

Most Processed Foods

Modern grocery stores often have over 40,000 products available on their shelves, and the vast majority of these products are some form of processed food. Processed foods comprise a good portion of what many Americans eat every day, and there is a wide variety of what these kinds of foods constitute. Heavily processed foods include most forms of prepackaged food, such as snack foods, crackers, chips, candy, and frozen pre-made meals. If you have any question about what constitutes a "processed food," you should assume that anything in a package with more than a few ingredients on the label is considered processed.

Often, these foods are high in ingredients like sugar and refined carbohydrates, which we should already be avoiding. Processed foods are most likely to include unnatural food additives, trans fats, preservatives, food dyes, GMO ingredients, and high amounts of added sodium (salt). Foods high in sodium, in particular, are something we should likely be avoiding as there is a link between elevated sodium intake and increased risk of cancer. (21) Many processed and preserved foods are too high in sodium, as are many fast foods, take-out foods, and foods you are served at a restaurant.

Pork

Pigs have an increased toxic load compared to other animals. This is due to the fact that they digest food very quickly, while also having reduced ability to eliminate toxins. These toxins accumulate in their flesh, and are transferred to us when we eat pork. It is not surprising that the Old Testament of the Bible instructs us to avoid pork. For these reasons, I advise avoiding pork and pork products completely. This includes ham, pork chops, bacon, sausage, pepperoni, hot dogs, and all other cured pork-based meats.

Shellfish

Shellfish include shrimp, lobster, crab, oysters, mussels, clams, and scallops. Leviticus 11:12 instructs us, "Whatever in the water does not have fins and scales is abhorrent to you." These scavengers can be thought of as oceanic vultures, searching the ocean floor for dead animals and other debris. As is the case with pigs, toxins accumulate, and anyone who eats these foods is also consuming these toxins. For these reasons, I recommend avoiding shellfish.

Trans Fats

Trans fats are man-made fats not found in nature. These are created by adding hydrogen to oils, and are used in order to prolong shelf life. They are present in shortening, margarine, and a wide variety of processed foods. They are denoted on labels as "hydrogenated oils" or "partially hydrogenated oils." We have known for quite some time that trans fats increase the risk of heart disease, despite the fact that they were touted for years as a better alternative to animal fats. They have been shown to increase certain kinds of cancer, as well. (22, 23)

Many food purveyors have sought to remove all forms of trans fats from their food, and these foods are now frequently labeled trans-fat free. Unfortunately, many are allowed to label their food as such, even if trace amounts can be found in those foods beneath a certain threshold. Since these types of fats are inherent only in processed foods, it is one more reason to avoid processed foods altogether.

Other Foods to Restrict

Sometimes, it is not the food itself, but how the food is prepared that can elevate its risk for promoting cancer. Fried foods are one instance of this. Anything fried is at the risk for becoming carcinogenic. (11) Meats that have been charred, smoked, overcooked, or cooked at extremely high temperatures can also contain carcinogenic compounds. (24) Basically, any foods which have been burned or left with grill marks should be avoided.

What Should We Have in Moderation?

Some foods are neither inherently good nor bad, and should instead be consumed in moderation. You might be surprised to learn that neither dairy nor alcohol have to be avoided completely, even if you are battling cancer. The key is to enjoy them in moderation, and to do so intelligently. The research does not support excluding them altogether. However, they are also not necessary, so if you choose to avoid them that is fine.

Alcohol

Alcohol is one substance which is often on the forbidden list when it comes to cancer. There are several proposed mechanisms for alcohol's relationship to cancer, including the formation of acetaldehyde, which is the result when the body breaks down alcohol. Acetaldehyde damages both DNA and proteins in the body. In addition, alcohol generates oxygen radicals, known as reactive oxygen species (ROS). Alcohol also slightly increases estrogen, which is linked to multiple cancers when present in the body in excess.

We know that heavy alcohol use is associated with increased risk of a variety of health issues, including cancer. However, the research on low-to-moderate alcohol intake and cancer is somewhat conflicting. One study found that light-to-moderate alcohol consumption (defined as up to one glass of wine per day for women, and up to two glasses of wine per day for men) is associated with a small but insignificant increase in risk of overall cancer. (25) The risk appears to be small, and not significant enough to justify complete avoidance in the setting of cancer prevention.

So what about alcohol in patients with cancer? Unfortunately, we do not have any solid studies on this topic, so I defer to common sense. Because alcohol does not provide any substantial anti-cancer benefits, it makes sense to restrict or avoid it if you have cancer. If you must have an alcoholic beverage while undergoing cancer treatment, you should limit it to 1 drink per week. One drink is equivalent to 5 ounces of wine, or 1.5 ounces of distilled spirits. Please ask your doctor if any alcohol consumption is allowed, as some alcoholic beverages can interact with certain chemotherapy agents.

Dairy

Dairy is another food group which may be enjoyed in limited amounts, but one which is certainly not necessary. Although dairy has been promoted for years as an important source of calcium, the small amount of calcium contained in dairy products can be easily obtained elsewhere in the diet or through supplementation. The concern with dairy as it relates to cancer is the common use of recombinant bovine growth hormone (rBGH) and antibiotics to produce larger cows and thus the amount of meat available for resale. We know that these additives not only harm the cows, but also affect the meat and milk from those cows as well. The resulting dairy products from these cows not only contain this same growth hormone and antibiotics, but also estrogens as well. Because multiple cancers are fueled by these additives, many in the alternative medical community recommend avoiding dairy altogether. This is especially true with respect to breast cancer, which is often stimulated by estrogen to grow and become more aggressive.

Studies on dairy products and cancer risk have largely been inconclusive, due to the fact that dairy is a large food group containing a wide variety of foods. (26) Regarding dairy consumption and breast cancer, one study reviewed 52 previous studies and concluded that there is no association between dairy product consumption and breast cancer risk. (27) Interestingly, another study found that women with breast cancer who consumed high fat dairy had a greater risk of death compared to those who consumed low fat dairy. (28)

I do not feel that dairy must be avoided completely if you enjoy it. When you do eat dairy, it is always best to eat organic, grass-fed dairy products without growth hormones. Goat dairy is preferable to cow dairy, but a small amount of cow dairy is still okay in moderation. I especially like grass-fed butter for its predominance of omega-3 fats, which are anti-inflammatory. Butter is very low in methionine, compared to other dairy products such as milk, yogurt, and cheese.

Eating Close to the Earth: What Foods Should We Focus On?

The foundation of my anti-cancer nutrition plan is eating as close to the earth as possible. What this means is that the focus of your diet should be foods that are mostly whole and unprocessed, and thus directly harvested from the earth. Eating this way means focusing on vegetables, fruits, whole grains, nuts, and seeds. Some healthy fats and animal protein, provided that they are from the proper sources, can be sprinkled in for good measure.

If you have cancer, you <u>must</u> eat a plant-based diet. The best way to go about shopping for a diet that is close to the earth is to shop around the perimeter of the grocery store; it is here where you will find fresh fruits, vegetables, legumes, and whole grains. Typically, I tell patients to avoid the aisles of a grocery store, because this is where you will find processed foods which offer little to no nutritional value. Certainly, some foods found in the aisles, such as nuts, nut butters, seeds, and extra virgin olive oils are perfectly fine to purchase. The idea of shopping around the perimeter should serve as a focal point, not a hard-and-fast rule.

Organic vs. Conventional

I believe that organic foods are far superior to non-organic foods. In the United States, the USDA organic label is what to look for; foods must meet a high standard before being issued this label, and as far as organic produce is concerned, the USDA organic label is the gold standard. Organic is best for a few reasons.

First, many of the harmful pesticides are not present in organic produce. It is important to note that many of the pesticides used in conventional farming are absorbed into the produce itself, meaning these chemicals will not simply wash off. While you should always wash organic produce before eating, the risk of contamination with potentially harmful pesticides is far lower with organic produce.

The standards of organic produce dictate that these foods cannot be genetically modified. There is much debate over whether such foods are safe to consume, but do we not want to err on the side of caution? While many regulatory bodies (and the companies that produce GMOs) insist that these foods are safe for consumption, we simply do not necessarily know what the long-term consequences are of eating a diet rich in genetically modified foods. Since purveyors are not required to label foods that are genetically modified, the organic label is a guarantee that what you are eating has not been genetically modified.

Finally, organic animal products are not tainted with the hormones and antibiotics routinely given to conventionally raised animals. This is an important difference if our goal is to prevent cancer. Some cancers have a strong hormonal component, and it is likely wise to avoid introducing unnatural and foreign hormones into our diet via animal products.

Raw vs. Cooked

Because we are focusing on food in its native form as much as possible, a logical question is, "Should I be eating raw foods?" The answer is, "Absolutely, yes!" Raw food is living food, preserved and unadulterated, as God intended it. Eating raw food provides numerous benefits, including the full amount of foods' nutrients and antioxidants. Raw, uncooked food also contains a significant portion of fiber.

Heating food alters it from its natural state, and in most cases, this reduces its nutritional value. In the case of fruits and vegetables, I recommend eating raw as much as possible. However, cooked produce is still extremely healthy, and is perfectly acceptable. I do not feel that an all-raw diet is necessary in most cases, nor is it practical.

Obviously, there are foods that we must cook in order to make them safer. Animal meat is a prime example of this. Please do not eat raw animal proteins, as they can contain bacteria, parasites, and other harmful organisms which are killed by cooking.

Vegetables

Vegetables, particularly green, leafy, and cruciferous vegetables such as spinach, kale, romaine, broccoli, Brussels sprouts, cabbage, and other vegetables should comprise a significant portion of what you consume on a daily basis. These vegetables are loaded with phytonutrients known to play a role in cancer prevention. (29) Cruciferous vegetables contain compounds known a glucosinolates, which are sulfuric compounds, which are also anti-cancer. Virtually all varieties of vegetables contain a wide palette of nutrients that provide a number of benefits, with a dual action of opposing cancer as well as nourishing healthy cells. For this reason, it is advised to "eat a rainbow," including a variety of colorful foods, as this will provide a wide spectrum of nutrients and antioxidants.

Some vegetables, such as beets, sweet potatoes and carrots are richer in naturally occurring sugars, and therefore have a higher glycemic index than other vegetables. However, these foods all have a rich nutrient content as well, and all have been shown to be protective against cancer. Carrots, in particular, have a higher glycemic index, but they can and should be consumed regularly for their known anti-cancer effects. Foods like these underscore our common-sense approach to crafting a diet that fights cancer.

Fruits

Like vegetables, fruits contain a wide variety of vital health-promoting nutrients which are beneficial in treating and preventing cancer. Fruits are higher in fructose—a naturally-occurring sugar—which means their glycemic index is higher than that of most vegetables. However, the naturally-occurring fiber in most fruits reduces the impact of sugar, meaning that the resulting glycemic rise and insulin spike are mitigated. This certainly makes consuming fruit much better than consuming refined carbohydrates or foods with added sugar.

Despite their higher sugar content, the benefits conferred by the broad spectrum of nutrients available in fruits makes them something we definitely want to include in our diet in high numbers. Particularly, fruits such as berries, apples, tomatoes, grapes, pineapples, and citrus fruits provide strong anti-cancer benefits. As with vegetables, attempt to eat a variety of colors in order to obtain a wide variety of nutrients and antioxidants.

What About Juicing?

Many anti-cancer plans recommend juicing. The main benefit of juicing is that it provides a very easily digestible form of fruits and vegetables, as it removes the harder-to-digest fiber. Another advantage of juicing is that it allows for a greater number of servings of fruits and vegetables each day.

Juicing is a valuable component of my anti-cancer nutrition plan. I feel that everyone benefits from juicing, especially when actively fighting cancer. Those with advanced cancer, including those who are having digestion issues with solid food, should obtain a significant portion of their calories from juicing.

An obvious criterion is that you should be making your own juices at home, with a juicer. This is NOT the same as a blender. A juicer is a special appliance that extracts the fiber, as opposed to a blender which simply pulverizes whatever is put into it. Both juicing and blending are acceptable, but for our purposes, juicing should be prioritized.

Buying store-bought juices, or simply ordering juice at a restaurant, is not acceptable. By juicing at home, you control what goes in your juice, which should only be organic fruits and vegetables. You will also benefit from knowing that your juice is fresh and contains the maximum number of beneficial components.

Here is a basic anti-cancer juice recipe I recommend for daily consumption:

- 8 carrots
- 8 celery stalks
- 1 green apple
- 1 beet

This makes a fairly large glass of juice, which can be consumed at once or gradually throughout the day. Contrary to popular belief, juice does not have to be consumed immediately after it is made in order to achieve the full benefits. I recommend storing any extra juice in mason jars in the refrigerator, and sipping on it throughout the day if not consuming it all at once. As mentioned previously, if you are actively fighting cancer, especially late-stage cancer, or are dealing with digestion issues, you will want to consume more than one serving of the above recipe each day. Some patients consume several of these per day. This amounts to a significant number of carrots. If your skin starts to turn orange, that is a clue that you are getting too many carotenoids and should back off. It is also not uncommon to notice some red streaks in your stool or urine as a result of the beets. I mention this only because it is often confused for blood.

There are many juice recipes, and I encourage you to experiment with various fruit and vegetable combinations. However, the above recipe contains a great collection of known anti-cancer foods. Feel free to add ginger, turmeric, lemon, lime, and even garlic to the above recipe if you desire.

You are probably wondering why I did not include leafy green vegetables. While these can be juiced, I have found that they do not produce much juice, and are best consumed in the form of a salad or a green smoothie.

Grains

When it comes to grains, our focus should be on whole, organic grains. Particularly, gluten-free grains such as oats, quinoa, buckwheat, and amaranth are okay in moderation. For those who tolerate gluten, the ancient grains and sprouted grains are acceptable in moderation as well.

Like fruit, the glycemic spike from grains is offset by the inherent fiber, which is why we focus on whole grains as opposed to processed grain products such as white flour. In white flour, the bran—the fiber and nutrient-containing portion of the grain—is removed, leaving only the starchy component. This starchy component is rich in carbohydrates, which prompts the insulin response seen in foods such as white breads or pastas. This is the reason why whole grains are considered healthier than refined grains. It is important to note that breads labeled "whole wheat" are not whole grain, and are still heavily processed. These should be avoided.

Nuts, Seeds, Oils, & Healthy Fats

Nuts and seeds are a good source of fiber, calories and healthy fats. They also contain some protein. Particularly, if you are undergoing treatment for cancer, the high caloric content of nuts and seeds can be a healthy source of calorically-dense food, thus preventing unwanted weight loss. Oils such as coconut, flax, and extra virgin olive oils also contain important cancer-fighting nutrients and constitute another excellent source of calories. Avocados are technically a fruit, but their fat content bears mentioning; they are a good source of healthy monounsaturated fat, among a variety of other nutrients. As mentioned previously, grass-fed butter is also a good option due to its healthy fat content.

Although we need some fat in the diet, we do not want a high fat diet. Studies have shown that cancer rates tend to be lower in countries which eat lower fat diets, however we do not know if this is causation or merely correlation. It is important to note that fat has been shown to increase metastasis and invasion. (30) Granted, this study was in mice, but it should prompt us to use caution in our fat consumption. We should focus on healthy types of fats, consumed in moderation and not in excess.

Protein

I recommend neither a low protein nor high protein diet. Moderation is key with protein; we want just enough to maintain a positive nitrogen balance, which is important for immune system function and maintaining muscle mass, but not so much protein that we overload the body and provide a hospitable environment for cancer. For most people, this amounts to approximately one gram of protein for every kilogram of body weight (1 kg = 2.2 lbs). For a 180 pound individual, this would be approximately 80 grams of protein daily. Vegetables and fruits are generally low in protein, so we must be intentional about obtaining protein from other sources.

Legumes, including beans, peas, and lentils, are good sources of protein (and fiber). Various nuts and seeds not only contain healthy fats, but some protein as well.

Although you should focus mostly on plants, it is not necessary to shun animal products altogether. Animal products can be enjoyed on my anti-cancer plan, however we do not want to eat these in excess since most animal proteins have high methionine. Free range eggs and beef, while not low in methionine, are lower than chicken, turkey, and fish.

In addition to methionine levels, another concern about meat is how it is sourced. Cows are a good example of this, as are other ruminants, such as bison and lamb. As ruminants, these animals' bodies are optimized for consuming grass. The design of their stomachs serves this purpose very well, and if these animals were found in the wild, they would eat grass exclusively.

Cows raised in the modern industrial era, however, are fed a diet mostly of corn and other foods unnatural to their diet. This is for a variety of reasons. Corn is a cheap feed product which allows a cow to put on weight quickly, particularly in the form of fat. The result is meat that is higher in fat but lower in overall nutrient content.

Some other things happen when cows are fed grass instead of corn. While the meat from these animals is often higher in fat, it is virtually void of beneficial, anti-inflammatory omega 3 fatty acids. Instead, the fat from conventionally raised cattle is high in inflammatory omega 6 fatty acids.

Omega 6 fatty acids, however, are not inherently bad. A good analogy would be the difference between eating an apple and eating high fructose corn syrup. Both contain sugar, but the way these two foods are metabolized by the body is very different. Similarly, not all omega 6 fats are equal. Some, in fact, can be very beneficial. In cows that are fed an unnatural diet, and given hormones and antibiotics, the inherent omega 6s are affected negatively, which renders them more inflammatory.

This is in contrast to cows fed their natural diet of grass. Not only does grass-fed meat become a good source of omega 3 fatty acids, they also contain a proper ratio of omega 3 to omega 6, and the inherent omega 6 fatty acids are of the beneficial variety. Grass-fed beef is also abundant in a variety of other nutrients, including beta carotene.

Small distinctions such as these go a long way when it comes to choosing the type of animal protein to include in your diet. Simply put, how your meat was raised and sourced matters. Grass-fed beef and bison, and pastured (free range) chickens and turkeys are much better options than their counterparts fed corn, grains, antibiotics, and growth hormones.

Fish can also be an excellent source of animal protein in the diet, although their methionine content is problematic. When eating fish, avoid bottom-feeding fish and crustaceans like catfish, oysters, mussels, lobster, and shrimp; these animals are much more likely to have accumulated environmental pollutants that subsequently contaminate their meat. Instead, focus on cold-water fish, such as salmon, tuna, and mackerel, as well as trout, cod, and halibut. Pollution is a significant source of concern with fish. When you do choose to eat fish, avoid the farm-raised varieties and opt for wild-caught.

Animal protein does not need to be eaten every day, nor should it be a focal point of your diet. I typically recommend that it be eaten no more than 2-3 times per week, provided it fits the aforementioned guidelines. This allows for some healthy animal protein, but not an excessive amount of methionine.

The Value of Herbs and Spices

One aspect of nutrition that is commonly overlooked is the inherent value of herbs and spices. Common herbs and spices include thyme, cinnamon, cloves, turmeric, cumin, oregano, sage, parsley, rosemary, mint, lavender, garlic, dill, cilantro, chives, and basil, among many others. There are a wide variety of herbs and spices that are known to provide some benefit against cancer, and we should certainly be using these liberally in our diet. (31, 32)

The diet that we have been discussing should be thought of less as a diet in the traditional sense, but more as a lifestyle. The diet I am recommending is not a diet you should "go on" for a period of time, but rather, it is a nutrition plan that should be maintained indefinitely. To this end, it is important to cultivate a diet that is flavorful, packed with nutrients, and yes, enjoyable!

For many people, making significant dietary changes can be difficult, because their tastes are so accustomed to highly processed foods, take-out meals, and fast foods as a large part of their diets. Many of these kinds of foods are heavily seasoned with manufactured flavoring agents like MSG, or high amounts of sodium and sugar, or loaded with fat. Truly, many people's taste buds become accustomed to the overpowering flavors inherent in many of today's convenience foods. Food purveyors know this; in fact, there is an active thrust to key in on addictive additives. When you have grown accustomed to these foods and flavors, changing your diet can literally mean breaking an addiction. It is not necessarily an easy task.

That said, eating a diet which is healthy and fights against cancer certainly does not mean a diet void of flavor. On the contrary, herbs and spices constitute a natural and healthy way to add real flavor to foods, the way people have been cooking for thousands of years. Not only are they beneficial for your health, they are also an important part of flavorful cooking.

Many herbs and spices, such as turmeric, garlic, and oregano, have shown such strong anti-cancer benefit (among other health benefits) that the importance of their liberal use in the kitchen cannot be overstated.

How Should My Plate Look?

Your plate should reflect the above principles, with a focus on organic, minimally processed foods, with a focus on plants. The vast majority of your plate—at least 50% of it—should consist of vegetables. These are foods such as spinach, broccoli, kale, Brussels sprouts, carrots, etc. Another 15% should contain fruits. Approximately 15% should contain a protein source such as legumes or animal protein. Another 15% should be grains. The final 5% should contain healthy fats.

These proportions do not have to be followed to the letter. However, for some individuals, it is helpful to visualize a plate when making decisions about the type and amount of food they eat. Do not feel that every meal has to fall into a perfect combination of foods. It is completely normal for some meals to contain more of one category of food than others. If you follow the basic principles we have discussed in this chapter, you will be fine.

Beverages

Water

Water should be your preferred beverage of choice. Strive to drink at least half of your bodyweight in ounces. For a person weighing 200 pounds, this would amount to 100 ounces of water per day. This ensures proper hydration, which is essential for optimal functioning of the body's cells, tissues, and organs. If you do not like water by itself, flavoring it with a wedge of lemon or lime is absolutely fine. Carbonated water, provided that it does not have added chemicals or artificial sweeteners, is okay in moderation. It is important to note that some people have issues digesting seltzer water, and in these cases, I recommend avoiding it.

The quality of your water is extremely important. Tap water contains additives which I have concerns about, the most notable of which is fluoride. A water filtration system is important. The commercial purifiers commonly available are not ideal, but they are better than nothing. A whole-house reverse water filtration system is ideal, as it not only filters drinking water, but also water used for bathing, washing hands, and laundry as well. Assume that all water consumed outside of your home, including at restaurants, is unfiltered.

I recommend drinking water throughout the day. Traditional Chinese medicine recommends drinking water between meals or meal courses, rather than with food, as this improves digestion. The thought is that food should be mixed only with saliva in order to be digested properly. I find this to be an intriguing idea, and one to explore if you are having any digestion or absorption issues. However, I realize that many people are in the habit of consuming water with their food, and breaking this habit can be a difficult one. I do not feel that avoiding water with meals should be a hard-and-fast rule.

Tea

There are a variety of teas, some of which are purported to possess anti-cancer properties. Green tea and Essiac tea are the two best known teas used in anti-cancer protocols. Green tea, known as Camellia sinensis, contains a substance called epigallocatechin-3-gallate, abbreviated EGCG. Research suggests that green tea plays a role in cancer prevention (33) and on suppressing cancer cell growth. (34)

Essiac tea contains a combination of herbs, most notably burdock root (Arctium lappa), Indian rhubarb (Rheum palmatum), slippery elm (Ulmus fulva), and sheep sorrel (Rumex acetosella). Although the individual components have been studied in isolation, there are no high quality studies on Essiac tea itself. A systematic review of all available literature found a lack of safety and efficacy data on Essiac formulations. (35)

I support the consumption of various herbal teas, including green tea, Essiac tea, and others. The only caution is that some teas, especially Essiac, should be consumed on an empty stomach as it can cause nausea, vomiting, and diarrhea if consumed with certain foods. However, we do not know how much tea should be consumed for a significant anti-cancer effect, and my suspicion is that it would require a lot of tea. This is not to say that consuming herbal teas is not beneficial for other reasons.

Coffee

Coffee is a very controversial and polarizing beverage as far as health is concerned. Some people say it is bad, others say it is good. The reason given for it being "bad" involves its reputation as an acidic food. However, as we have mentioned before, the pH of a specific food or drink is largely inconsequential in terms of its health potential in the body. There have also been concerns in the past about caffeine, and whether or not it is harmful.

There are now multiple studies on coffee (the natural, caffeinated version) and cancer. One study found that coffee reduces risk for brain cancer by 40%. (36) Another study found that at least 2 cups of coffee a day reduce colon cancer risk. (37) Yet another study found that at least 3 cups of coffee daily prevent or delay the onset of certain types of cancer in women, including breast, colon, lung, and ovarian. (38)

I feel that coffee is quite beneficial for those with cancer, as well as those wanting to prevent it. The anti-cancer benefits seem to occur with at least 3 cups of coffee per day, and in some studies, 4 or more. You should consume the caffeinated version, as the decaffeinated version typically adds some harmful chemicals to the process. As with all other foods, organic is preferred. Ideally, you should drink your coffee black, but if you must add cream, use it sparingly and try to use organic cream. If you require a sweetener, opt for a natural sweetener such as stevia.

Cancer Nutrition: Summary of Recommendations

- Eliminate added sugar, which is cancer's preferred (but not only!) fuel source. The only sugar you should be consuming is that found naturally in fruits, vegetables, legumes, and grains.

- Minimize the amino acid methionine, as it has been shown in studies to be required for cancer cell growth. This means that a majority of the diet will be plant-based.

- Prioritize organic fruits and vegetables. Experiment with a wide variety of foods here, and "eat the rainbow." Vegetables should predominate over fruits, and raw food should take precedence over cooked food. Eat organic whenever possible.

- Animal protein should be limited. When choosing animal protein sources, avoid mass produced meats, and instead opt for more natural sources including free range eggs and grass-fed beef. Eggs and beef have less methionine than fish and chicken.

- Limit daily protein intake to approximately 1 gram of protein per kilogram of bodyweight. To calculate this number, divide your body weight in pounds by 2.2. This is your body weight in kilograms, and is the number of grams of protein you should strive for. This provides enough protein to help maintain muscle mass and for bodily processes, but not so much that we worry about creating an overly anabolic (growth-promoting) environment.

- Don't forget about legumes, including beans, lentils, and peas. They offer a wide range of benefits, including protein and fiber.

- Eat grains such as oats, quinoa, buckwheat, and amaranth. Ancient grains, including the sprouted variety, are excellent. Otherwise, gluten should be limited. Consume no white flour, such as those found in most breads, cereals, and pastas.

- Have some healthy fats, especially those from natural sources such as avocados, coconuts, olives, nuts, and seeds. Medium chain triglyceride (MCT) oil and grass-fed butter are both excellent sources as well.

- Avoid white sugar and high fructose corn syrup, as well as artificial sweeteners such as sucralose (Splenda) and aspartame (Equal). Instead, opt for a natural sweetener such as stevia. The jury is still out on xylitol and erythritol, but I feel that these are okay in moderation.
- Drink plenty of water. A good goal is to drink half of your bodyweight in ounces. A 150-pound person should drink at least 75 ounces of water each day, mostly between meals. Sodas and sports drinks should be avoided.
- Coffee and tea are encouraged, as they both have anti-cancer effects. Organic is best.

When making the above changes, your body (and mind) might take time to adjust. The carbohydrate and sugar cravings can be powerful at times, and have been likened by some to those of a drug addict going through withdrawals. Headaches, fatigue, and irritability are not uncommon, and typically last anywhere from a few days to 1-2 weeks. However, these symptoms (if they occur at all) are not permanent. In fact, once you undergo this transition phase, you will find that you feel better, with improved energy and better focus. Decide now to make these changes a lifestyle, rather than merely a diet. The former is something you can do long-term, whereas the latter implies only a short-term commitment.

If all of this seems daunting, please keep in mind that what you eat makes a significant difference! A large study in the Journal of Clinical Oncology found that women with breast cancer who ate five or more servings of vegetables and fruit each day, and exercised for 30 minutes per day six days per week, cut their risk of dying in half in the first two years following their diagnosis. (39) If that were a patentable drug, every oncologist would prescribe it to their patients, and our cancer treatment outcomes would be far superior to what they currently are!

Fasting

Once your body is accustomed to the above plan (at least 1-2 weeks), I highly recommend incorporating fasting. In addition to the Biblical basis for fasting, we now have scientific evidence that fasting reduces inflammation and stimulates the immune system. There are also studies showing that fasting reduces multiple chemotherapy-induced side effects. (40)

There are several ways to incorporate fasting, including daily fasting and block fasting. Daily fasting entails fasting every day, while block fasting entails fasting only certain days in succession each week or month. I prefer daily fasting, referred to as intermittent fasting. This method utilizes a specific fasting period and eating window each day. Because we wake up in a fasted state, I like to extend this fasting period into the day. For most people, skipping breakfast and waiting until lunchtime or early afternoon to eat works well. I recommend an eating window of approximately 8 hours per day, which leaves a 16-hour fasting period. For example:

- Eating window: 12:00 PM until 8:00 PM
- Fasting window: 8:01 PM until 11:59 AM

This can be adjusted according to your specific schedule. For example, if you really like breakfast, your eating window could be 7:00 AM until 3:00 PM.

I have found that an 8-hour eating window allows enough time to consume a healthy and well-rounded diet, but also plenty of time for fasting. During the fasting period, you are not to consume any calories. Many people enjoy a water fast, which entails consuming only water while fasting. Others will also include coffee and herbal tea, sweetened with stevia if necessary. For some people, easing into fasting by only prolonging the fasting window an hour or two at first will be necessary.

Something magical happens during the fasting window! Studies have shown that fasting not only reduces chemotherapy side effects, but also suppresses tumor progression and improves prognosis. (41) Of course, further research on fasting and cancer needs to be performed, but at this point I feel that most patients can benefit from fasting.

Please note that fasting should not be used by patients who are malnourished, undernourished, underweight, or nutritionally depleted. In these cases, frequent feedings throughout the day are essential, and fasting would likely cause more harm than good. For those who feel they are good candidates for fasting, doing so under the supervision of a trained healthcare professional is essential.

Dr. Stegall's Seven Superfoods

Although there are hundreds of amazing foods from which to choose, there are some which stand out as "superfoods." Here are my top seven:

1. Garlic

Garlic is perhaps the most anti-cancer food in existence. While we associate garlic with its characteristic smell and taste, it turns out that this member of the alliaceous family is a powerful cancer fighter. Studies have shown that garlic helps prevent cancer, and also kills multiple cancer cell lines. One study examined the abilities of over 30 vegetable extracts to inhibit the growth of a variety of cancer cell types, and garlic completely halted the growth of all cancers. (42) I recommend using fresh garlic liberally on salads, in sautéed vegetables, and with any other foods you like.

If you do not like garlic, other vegetables from the Allium family also have anti-cancer properties. These include green onions, yellow onions, and leeks.

2. Broccoli

Broccoli is a cruciferous vegetable which contains sulforaphane and indole-3-carbinol (I3C), two especially potent substances with cancer-fighting properties. Sulforaphane has been studied extensively, and is especially important to us because it targets cancer stem cells (CSCs). (43)

Broccoli is best eaten raw, but if you do not like the texture, it is perfectly fine to steam it. However, do not boil it or microwave it, as the anti-cancer properties are neutralized, and you will not derive nearly as much of the cancer-fighting benefits of broccoli. Broccoli sprouts are another way to get these powerful anti-cancer benefits.

Other cruciferous vegetables include Brussels sprouts, cauliflower, kale, and red cabbage. These are also powerful anti-cancer foods you should eat, although none contain as much sulforaphane as broccoli.

3. Carrots

High in carotenoids such as alpha- and beta-carotene, as well as bioflavonoids, carrots pack a serious anti-cancer punch. Studies have shown that carrots kill cancer cells, reduce inflammation, and improve immune system function. (44) Carrots are great to eat by themselves as a snack, or as a key part of a juicing regimen.

4. Beets

Also known as red beetroot, beets derive their characteristic red color from betalain, which has been shown to starve tumors and hinder cell division. Beets have also been found in studies to display a direct cancer cell killing behavior. (45)

5. Ginger

Ginger has been shown to kill various types of cancer cells in lab studies. As an added bonus, it has been shown to modulate the expression of cancer genes, scavenge for free radicals, and induce apoptosis of cancer cells. (46) As an added bonus, ginger also helps settle the gut and ease digestion, and is my favorite natural treatment for nausea.

Because ginger is sweet, it can be added to herbal teas or used to top oatmeal or sweet potatoes. It is also a great addition to carrot and beet juice.

6. Tomatoes

Although commonly thought of as vegetables, tomatoes are actually fruits. Their anti-cancer effect comes from lycopene, a carotenoid that gives tomatoes their bright red color. Lycopene is well-documented for its ability to prevent cancer (47), however, it has also been shown to have a cytotoxic effect.

Tomatoes should be enjoyed on salads and in homemade sauces and salsas, or simply eaten by themselves.

7. Cranberries

Cranberries contain ellagic acid as well as polyphenols, both of which have been shown to inhibit the growth of tumors. Cranberries specifically have a high number of anthocyanidins and proanthocyanidins, polyphenols that are especially anti-cancer. One particular study investigated the ability of various fruits to reduce oxidative damage and also slow the proliferation of cancer, and cranberries were the clear winner in both categories. (48) Cranberries are a great addition to oatmeal, smoothies, or simply eaten alone as a snack.

Cranberries are not the only berry with anti-cancer attributes. Blueberries, strawberries, raspberries, and blackberries also have many valuable properties and should ideally be included in your diet as well.

These seven foods should be a regular—if not daily—part of your nutrition regimen. I highly recommend you eat these foods as often as you can! And of course, be sure to freely use herbs and spices to season your foods. The collective anti-cancer effect contained within this approach comprises a powerful tool in our arsenal.

(1) Garber JE, Offit K. Hereditary cancer predisposition syndromes. J Clin Oncol 2005; 23(2): 276-92.

(2) Song M, Giovannucci E. Preventable Incidence and Mortality of Carcinoma Associated With Lifestyle Factors Among White Adults in the United States. JAMA Oncol 2016; 2(9): 1154-61.

(3) Collective, The Tincture. "Nutrition and Cancer: Where do we go from here? – Tincture." Tincture, Tincture, 4 Mar. 2016, tincture.io/nutrition-and-cancer-where-do-we-go-from-here-7f93632e0464. Accessed 21 Aug. 2017.

(4) Johnson SB, Park HS, Gross CP, et al. Use of alternative medicine for cancer and its impact on survival. J Natl Cancer Inst 2018; 110(1): 121-4.

(5) Diet, Nutrition, and Cancer Directions for Research. National Academy Press, 1983.

(6) McCleary L. Feed Your Brain, Lose Your Belly. Austin: Greenleaf Book Group Press, 2011. Print.

(7) "Generally Recognized as Safe – But Is It?" EWG, Nov. 2014, www.ewg.org/research/ewg-s-dirty-dozen-guide-food-additives/generally-recognized-as-safe-but-is-it#.Wl6Oj62ZORs.

(8) "Department of Animal Science - Plants Poisonous to Livestock." Cornell University Department of Animal Science, poisonousplants.ansci.cornell.edu/toxicagents/aflatoxin/aflatoxin.html.

(9) Center for Food Safety and Applied Nutrition. "Public Health Focus - Bisphenol A (BPA): Use in Food Contact Application." U S Food and Drug Administration Home Page, Center for Food Safety and Applied Nutrition, www.fda.gov/newsevents/publichealthfocus/ucm064437.htm#summary.

(10) Stern V. "Does BPA Increase Cancer Risk." Medscape, 4 Mar. 2015, www.medscape.com/viewarticle/840559.

(11)   "Known and Probable Human Carcinogens." American Cancer Society, www.cancer.org/cancer/cancer-causes/general-info/known-and-probable-human-carcinogens.html.

(12)   "About RbGH." Center for Food Safety, www.centerforfood safety.org/issues/1044/rbgh/about-rbgh.

(13)   Allen BG, Bhatia SK, Anderson CM, et al. Ketogenic diets as an adjuvant cancer therapy: History and potential mechanism. Redox Biol 2014; 2: 963-70.

(14)   Bhatia T. "10 Most Common GMO Foods To Avoid." Food Matters, 19 Nov. 2017, www.foodmatters.com/article/10-most-common-gmo-foods.

(15)   Freeman HJ. Malignancy in adult celiac disease. World J Gastroenterol 2009; 15(13): 1581.

(16)   Ap. "Just How Much Sugar Do Americans Consume? It's Complicated." CBS News, CBS Interactive, 20 Sept. 2016, www.cbsnews.com/news/just-how-much-sugar-do-americans-consume-its-complicated/.

(17)   Sugimura T, Birnbaum SM, Winitz M, et al. Quantitative nutritional studies with water-soluble, chemically defined diets. VIII. The forced feeding of diets each lacking in one essential amino acid. Arch Biochem Biophys 1959; 81(2): 448-55.

(18)   Halpern BC, Clark BR, Hardy DN, et al. The effect of replacement of methionine by homocysteine on survival of malignant and normal adult mammalian cells in culture. Proc Natl Acad Sci USA 1974; 71(4): 1133-6.

(19)   Breillout F, Antoine E, Poupon MF. Methionine dependency of malignant tumors: a possible approach for therapy. J Natl Cancer Inst 1990; 82(20): 1628-32.

(20)   Guo HY, Herrera H, Groce A, et al. Expression of the biochemical defect of methionine dependence in fresh patient tumors in primary histoculture. Cancer Res 1993; 53(11): 2479-83.

(21) Wang XQ. Review of salt consumption and stomach cancer risk: Epidemiological and biological evidence." World J Gastroenterol 2009; 15(18): 2204.

(22) "Trans Fats May Increase Risk." Breastcancer.org, www. breastcancer.org/research-news/20080411b.

(23) Slattery ML, et al. "Trans-fatty acids and colon cancer. Nutr Cancer 2001; 39(2): 170-5.

(24) "Chemicals in Meat Cooked at High Temperatures and Cancer Risk." National Cancer Institute, www.cancer.gov/about-cancer/ causes-prevention/risk/diet/cooked-meats-fact-sheet.

(25) Car Y, Willett WC, Rimm EB, et al. Light to moderate intake of alcohol, drinking patterns, and risk of cancer: results from two prospective US cohort studies. BMJ 2015; 351: h4238.

(26) Lampe JW. Dairy products and cancer. J Am Coll Nutr 2011; 30(5 Suppl 1): 464S-70S.

(27) Parodi PW. Dairy product consumption and the risk of breast cancer. J Am Coll Nutr 2005; 24(6 Suppl): 556S-68S.

(28) Kroenke CH, Kwan ML, Sweeney C, et al. High- and low-fat dairy intake, recurrence, and mortality after breast cancer diagnosis. J Natl Cancer Inst 2013; 105(9): 616-23.

(29) Higdon J, et al. Cruciferous Vegetables and Human Cancer Risk: Epidemiologic Evidence and Mechanistic Basis. Pharmacol Res 2007; 55(3): 224-36.

(30) Pascual G, Avgustinova A, Mejetta S, et al. Targeting metastasis-initiating cells through the fatty acid receptor CD36. Nature 2017; 541: 41-5.

(31) Kaefer CM, Milner JA. The Role of Herbs and Spices in Cancer Prevention. J Nutr Biochem 2008; 19(6): 347-61.

(32) Kaefer CM, Milner JA. "Herbs and Spices in Cancer Prevention and Treatment." Herbal Medicine: Biomolecular and Clinical Aspects., 2nd ed., CRC Press/Taylor & Francis, 2011.

(33) Liu J, Xing J, and Fei Y. Green tea (Camellia sinensis) and cancer prevention: a systematic review of randomized trials and epidemiological studies. Chin Med 2008; 3: 12.

(34) Zhao T, Sun Q, del Rincon SV, ,et al. Gallotannin imposes S phase arrest in breast cancer cells and suppresses the growth of triple negative tumors in vivo. PLoS One 2014; 9(3): e92853.

(35) Ulbricht C, Weissner W, Hashmi S, et al. Essiac: systematic review by the natural standard research collaboration. J Soc Integr Oncol 2009; 7(2): 73-80.

(36) Holick CN, Smith SG, Giovannucci E, et al. Coffee, tea, caffeine intake, and risk of adult glioma in three prospective cohort studies. Cancer Epidemiol Biomarkers Prev 2010; 19(1): 39-47.

(37) Oba S, Shimizu N, Nagata C, et al. The relationship between the consumption of meat, fat, and coffee and the risk of colon cancer: a prospective study in Japan. Cancer Letters 2006; 244 (2): 260-7.

(38) Lukic M, Licaj I, Lund E, et al. Coffee consumption and the risk of cancer in the Norwegian Women and Cancer (NOWAC) Study. Eur J Epidemiol 2016; 31(9): 905-16.

(39) Pierce JP, Sefanick ML, Flatt SW, et al. Greater survival after breast cancer in physically active women with high vegetable-fruit intake regardless of obesity. J Clin Oncol 2007; 25(17): 2345-51.

(40) Safdie FM, Dorff T, Quinn D, et al. Fasting and cancer treatment in humans: a case series report. Aging (Albany NY) 2009; 1(12): 988-1007.

(41) Sun L, Li YJ, Yang X, et al. Effect of fasting therapy in chemotherapy-protection and tumor-suppression: a systematic review. Transl Cancer Res 2017; 6(2): 354-65.

(42) Boivin D, Lamy S, Lord-Dufour S, et al. Antiproliferative and antioxidant activities of common vegetables: A comparative study. *Food Chemistry* 2009; 112: 374-80.

(43) Li Y, Zhang T. Targeting cancer stem cells with sulforaphane, a dietary component from broccoli and broccoli sprouts. *Future Oncol* 2013; 9(8): 1097-1103.

(44) da Silva Dias J. Nutritional and Health Benefits of Carrots and Their Seed Extracts. *Food and Nutr Sci* 2014; 5: 2147-56.

(45) Kapadia GJ, Azuine MA, Rao GS, et al. Cytotoxic effect of the red beetroot (Beta vulgaris L.) extract compared to doxorubicin (Adriamycin) in the human prostate (PC-3) and breast (MCF-7) cancer cell lines. *Anticancer Agents Med Chem* 2011; 11(3): 280-4.

(46) Baliga MS, Haniadka R, Pereira MM, et al. Update on the chemopreventative effects of ginger and its phytochemicals. *Crit Rev Fod Sci Nutr* 2011; 51(6): 499-523.

(47) Dahan K, Fennal M, Kumar NB. Lycopene in the prevention of prostate cancer. *J Soc Integr Oncol* 2008; 6(1): 29-36.

(48) Sun J, Chu YF, Wu X, and Liu RH. Antioxidant and antiproliferative activities of common fruits. *J Agric Food Chem* 2002; 50(25): 7449-54.

CHAPTER 7

Supplementation in Cancer Prevention and Treatment

"Nutritional supplements are not a substitute
for a nutritionally balanced diet."
– Deepak Chopra, MD

The Role of Specific Supplements

According to Dr. Google, there are many nutritional supplements which have an anti-cancer effect, to the point that a lot of people feel that they can build an effective cancer fighting regimen with supplements alone. However, supplements are not intended to be a stand-alone treatment. They are called "supplements" for a reason! With that said, supplements can be a very valuable adjunct to the other treatments we employ, provided we use them correctly.

There are several questions we must ask ourselves about any potential supplement:

1. Does it work? In other words, do we have scientific evidence for its anti-cancer effect, and if so, is it high quality evidence? Human

studies are much more meaningful than a study on lab rats or on cells in the lab. But even lab studies are more meaningful than an online testimonial, especially if that testimonial is featured on a website selling the supplement.

2. Does it have any known side effects, contraindications, or interactions? Many people believe that because a supplement is "natural," that it cannot possibly have any negative side effects. This is a very dangerous belief. Any substance, even a natural one, which has a positive effect in the body also has the potential for a negative effect. There are many documented side effects from supplements when an inappropriate amount is taken. There are also numerous examples of supplements interacting with other supplements or pharmaceuticals. Finally, some supplements are contraindicated in patients with certain issues, such as kidney or liver disease.

3. Is it of good quality? Although there are certain standards in place for supplement manufacturers, there exists a great deal of leeway in terms of the quality and purity of the components of a supplement. I cannot stress enough the importance of obtaining high quality supplements. You are likely to be disappointed by the quality of what you will find on the shelves of your local pharmacy or big box retailer. Also, be careful of what you find online, as it could have little to none of the components it is supposed to have. The ideal approach is to go through an integrative physician who not only understands how a wide variety of supplements work, but also has access to practitioner-only supplements which abide by the highest standards of quality, purity, and research.

As with any other treatment, I believe that supplements should be individualized for each patient. A one-size-fits-all approach rarely works. In addition, we must be very cognizant of the other therapies we are employing, including pharmaceuticals, and possible interactions. More is not always better. Remember, the key is not simply what you take, but what your body is able to digest and absorb.

Because supplements should be individualized for each patient, it would be inappropriate and irresponsible for me to list all potential supplements I use with my patients. However, there are definitely some supplements that I recommend for a majority of my patients. As is the case with diet, the main goal of supplements is to create an internal terrain that makes cancer development very difficult, with perhaps some cancer cell killing as an added benefit. The following list of supplements constitutes those which I feel are foundational. Some are intended to "alter the terrain" by improving the body's function in some way and/or reduce the chances that cancer can grow and thrive. Others are intended to provide a true anti-cancer effect by directly killing cancer cells.

Baking Soda

Recall that cancer thrives in an acidic (low pH) environment. These acidic conditions do not cause cancer, but rather, are caused by cancer. Thus, the thinking that an acidic pH causes cancer and that an alkaline pH prevents cancer is unfounded. However, because cancer, once formed, creates an acidic environment around the tumor, and since this acidic environment stimulates the growth and progression of cancer, increasing the pH (alkalization) of the tumor microenvironment sounds like a great idea. Despite the popularity of so-called "alkaline diets," we cannot accomplish this through dietary measures. In fact, recent studies have concluded that alkaline diets and alkaline water are not supported by research and that their promotion to treat or prevent cancer is unjustified. (1) Thus, baking soda is not an effective alkalinizing agent.

However, research has shown that cancer cells have pH sensors on their cell membranes which stimulate downstream effects including migration and metastasis. Baking soda has been shown to alter these sensors, thereby disrupting these signals. (2) Further research confirmed these findings. (3) Although we do not have any large scale human studies on baking soda and cancer treatment, research thus far has been encouraging. A study done on mice with metastatic breast cancer found that mice who received baking soda water had significantly greater survival than those that did not. (4)

In addition, baking soda also seems to aid in healthy detoxification and perhaps even reduces resistance to chemotherapy agents. Finally, it has the advantage of being a nutritional therapy that patients can easily and inexpensively do at home. I recommend that patients take 1 teaspoon of Bob's Red Mill Baking Soda three times per day between meals. It should be taken 30 minutes before eating, and two hours after eating, to avoid negatively impacting digestion (we want an acidic stomach to optimize digestion, and baking soda, as an alkaline substance, alters that acidic environment). It is best to mix the baking soda with 8-12 ounces of purified water. In addition, 1-2 teaspoons of fresh lemon juice can be added as well, for taste as well as additional alkalization. Apple cider vinegar can be used in place of lemon juice, if desired.

The baking soda protocol can be taken alone, but also pairs very well with my recommendations in the nutrition chapter.

Beta-1,3D Glucan

Beta glucan is a supplement which I include in all of my cancer treatment protocols. Beta glucans help form the structural walls of yeast, fungi, and seaweed. They are what we refer to as biological response modifiers, due to their wide range of effects in the body including immunity against infectious agents as well as a reduction in oxidative stress. (5) There is evidence that beta glucan is effective against multiple cancer types. (6, 7), and research is pointing toward it likely being beneficial for all cancers, especially when combined with vitamin C and resveratrol. (8)

The beta glucan I use with my patients is the Transfer Point beta-1,3D Glucan, from Better Way Health. This is a well-researched, highly potent formula which I cannot recommend highly enough. The anti-cancer dose is one 500 mg capsule per 50 pounds of body weight daily. Thus, a 200-pound individual would take 4 capsules daily. For prevention purposes, I recommend one capsule per day. I take it myself for immune system health.

Curcumin/Turmeric

Curcumin is the active component of turmeric, which is of course a spice. There have been numerous studies on curcumin's benefit against cancer, though many thus far have only been done on cancer cell lines. The human studies we do have provide good evidence that curcumin has some benefit against cancer. (9) Curcumin is thought to inhibit some of the genes that promote cancer cell growth. Curcumin is also known to reduce inflammation, which is a key factor in cancer's development. As an active component of turmeric, supplementing with curcumin constitutes a convenient way of obtaining therapeutic amounts. A typical anti-cancer dose is 4-5 grams (4000-5000 mg) per day. I have a high quality one manufactured for use with my patients. Supplementing with curcumin should be in addition to liberal use of turmeric and other spices for cooking and seasoning.

Of note, curcumin is a mild blood thinner and should be used with caution in patients taking pharmaceutical blood thinners, or who are having surgery in the near future.

Digestive Enzymes

"You are what you eat," is a common saying, but "you are what you digest and absorb," would be a more accurate statement. Digestion begins in the mouth, and continues as we move into the stomach and small intestine. Enzymes are responsible for breaking down proteins into their constituent amino acids, carbohydrates into sugars, and fats into fatty acids. The body produces its own digestive enzymes, but in many cases, we become deficient. This deficiency results in decreased digestion and absorption of key nutrients, as well as symptoms of poor digestion including acid reflux, bloating, nausea, vomiting, diarrhea, and constipation, to name a few.

For many individuals, I recommend a well-rounded digestive enzyme supplement at the start of each meal. The formulation should include amylase, lipases, and proteases so that carbohydrates, fats, and proteins, respectively, will be broken down properly. Individuals who are not having any digestive symptoms can probably get away with a lower dose, or perhaps even avoid digestive enzyme supplementation altogether. However, given the prevalence of digestive issues in society today, completely asymptomatic individuals are few and far between.

EGCG

Epigallocatechin-3-gallate, more commonly referred to as EGCG, is a well-studied antioxidant that is a component of green tea. Several studies in vivo and in vitro have confirmed that EGCG can reduce cancer risk, might protect against metastasis, and likely protects against angiogenesis. (10) Many patients would opt to simply drink a lot of green tea throughout the day, which is certainly fine. However, like turmeric, EGCG is only one component of green tea. Supplementing with EGCG is a sure way to get the therapeutic benefits of this particular antioxidant.

The best, and most researched, green tea supplement is Capsol-T. The supplement has to be taken every 4 hours, including overnight. Because this was less than ideal, the company made a sustained-release version for use overnight. The recommended combination is to take the normal version throughout the day, and the sustained-release overnight. One capsule is equivalent to drinking 16 cups of green tea, but without the caffeine or liquid.

Essential Fatty Acids

Many people today are aware of omega 3 fats, which are the healthy, anti-inflammatory essential fats. These omega 3s are important to counter the inflammatory environment in the body which results from all of the stressors and toxins to which we are exposed. In an attempt to get plenty of omega 3s, a significant number of people take fish oil supplements. However, I believe that there is a much better way.

Recall that Dr. Otto Warburg's research over 70 years ago uncovered the fact that cancer is a result of oxygen deprivation inside the cell. (11) He also stated that the distinguishing factor between a benign, non-cancerous cell and a malignant, cancerous cell was the duration of the oxygen deficit. (12) Dr. Brian Peskin, a prominent researcher on fatty acids, has found that fats are best acquired from their native source—termed parent essential oils or parent essential fatty acids. He states that fish oils, in addition to being highly processed with chemicals and toxic derivatives, do not contain enough of these parent essential fatty acids. (13) By obtaining parent essential fatty acids in the form such as that found in coconut oil, flax oil, sunflower oil, evening primrose oil, and pumpkin oil, the correct type of fatty acids are obtained. These parent essential oils—in contrast to their fish oil counterparts—are powerful oxygen carriers.

Dr. Peskin's research has determined that the proper ratio of parent omega 6s to parent omega 3s needed by the body is between 1:1 and 4:1. This is contrary to what most people believe. We have been told for years that omega 6s are bad, because they cause inflammation, and omega 3s are good, because they are anti-inflammatory. However, it is important to note that only adulterated omega 6s, such as those found in processed foods, cause inflammation. Parent omega 6s, as found in their native plant-based form, do not. In fact, parent omega 6s are quite anti-inflammatory, by virtue of the fact that they are capable of carrying much more oxygen than parent omega 3s.

Contrary to many integrative physicians, I do not recommend fish oil supplements. Rather, I recommend a supplement of parent essential fatty acids, which I have manufactured for my patients in my practice.

Probiotics

I recommend probiotics for virtually all of my patients, but they are likely a supplement everyone should be on regardless of cancer status. Probiotics are not an anti-cancer supplement, per se, but they are an excellent supplement for systemic health. The role of probiotics is simply to replace and support the beneficial bacteria colonies inherent in the gut and to balance the terrain therein.

There is mounting evidence that good gut health has tremendous benefits for immunity and for the brain. Unfortunately, because of poor diets, stressful lifestyles, and the general "toxic soup" in which we all live, the beneficial strains of bacteria can become damaged or depleted. Problems such as leaky gut are commonplace, and as a result, we are exposed to a greater number of pathogens than we otherwise would be. This has been shown to stimulate the immune system in a negative way, which paves the way for the variety of autoimmune diseases that are so prevalent today. Some theories regarding cancer are that it is actually an autoimmune disease.

Probiotics are a good supplement to take to support overall health; remember, the chief goal of diet and supplements is to create an internal terrain that makes it difficult for cancer to survive, or even develop in the first place. For most patients, a high dose probiotic is in order—at least 30 billion colony forming units (CFUs). For most of my patients, I put them on a 100 billion CFU supplement which I have made to my specifications. I have patients take it daily. Those with more significant digestive issues will need to be on an even higher strength probiotic for a few weeks, on the order of 200-250 billion CFUs, after which I will transition them to the 100 billion CFU probiotic.

Because I know some will ask: simply eating yogurt is not the same thing, and will not make a difference in terms of adding beneficial gut bacteria.

Resveratrol

Resveratrol is a polyphenol which is naturally occurring in grapes and berries. Interestingly, plants produce it in response to various stressors, including infection, ultraviolet radiation, and mechanical injury. (15) Resveratrol is purported to have many beneficial properties of interest to us as an anti-cancer agent, including direct cancer cell killing, being anti-inflammatory, and even protecting healthy cells during chemotherapy.

Unfortunately, a significant portion of clinical studies on resveratrol have been in vitro studies on cancer cell lines. Not surprisingly, the results of these studies have been promising. In addition, animal studies have shown an anti-cancer effect of resveratrol. However, there have not been many clinical studies involving humans, and the results thus far have been mixed. (16)

Resveratrol's effects have been shown to be dose-dependent. (17) For anti-cancer purposes, I typically use a trans-resveratrol supplement manufactured for my patients, at a total daily dose of 400-800 mg daily. This is typically divided into a morning and evening dose.

Selenium

One of the most important micronutrients is selenium. Also known as a trace mineral, selenium deficiency has been established as a risk factor for developing cancer. (18) Another study found that individuals supplementing with selenium reduced their risk of cancer by 24%. The cancer prevention effect improved even more in those individuals who were selenium deficient; supplementing with selenium in these patients reduced cancer risk by 36%! (19)

Selenium has also shown an anti-cancer effect in vitro and in vivo. The main action of selenium against cancer involves altering the regulatory elements within cancer cells, signaling to the immune system that they are foreign and must be eliminated. (20) This explains why it causes such a significant reduction in cancer risk in those who supplement with it. In addition, selenium has also been proposed as an anti-metastatic agent via multiple mechanisms, including an inhibition of cancer cell motility as well as by stimulating a reduction in angiogenic factors. (21) It also reduces oxidative stress, improves detoxification, and helps the body eliminate metals.

The anti-cancer dose of selenium is 200-400 mcg daily. A supplement is typically the easiest way to achieve this amount. However, I have found selenium to be an excellent component of my intravenous (IV) protocols.

Brazil nuts have a high amount of selenium (approximately 120 mcg of selenium per nut), but they are prohibitively high in methionine so I do not recommend that cancer patients consume them.

Vitamin D3

There have been many studies conducted on vitamin D, and subsequently many theories about optimal levels. When we test for vitamin D, we are testing for levels of 25 hydroxy vitamin D (usually listed as 25-OH vitamin D on a lab report). Some studies have suggested a blood level of 40-60 ng/mL of vitamin D is ideal, others suggested 50-70 ng/mL, and others suggested 80-100 ng/mL. Current studies show that for anti-cancer purposes, it is optimal to keep vitamin D levels in the 50-70 range.

This is a very important point, because it involves a portion of the body's immune system known as T helper cells. These cells can be thought of as a movie director, or a symphony conductor, directing the immune system to function in specific ways. There are two types of T helper cells, known as Th1 and Th2. The Th1 cells govern what is known as cell-mediated immunity, involving immune cells such as natural killer cells and others. These cells are important for protecting the immune system, especially in patients receiving chemotherapy. (22) Optimizing the 25-OH vitamin D in this 50-70 ng/mL range results in a Th1 dominant immune system.

When 25-OH vitamin D levels exceed 70 ng/mL, we shift the immune system from Th1 dominance to Th2 dominance. When we have Th2 dominance, this is the humoral, or antibody-mediated, immune response. Although Th2 dominance results in less inflammation, it also causes more allergic responses and is much less supportive of a strong immune system.

Vitamin D is an example of how more is not always better. Regardless, most people who do not supplement with vitamin D are typically below 20 ng/mL on a 25-OH vitamin D blood level. It is rare to see someone who can simply spend time in the sun and get enough vitamin D. With supplementation, it is typically easy to get patients to optimal levels of vitamin D. For virtually all patients, a well-absorbed vitamin D3 supplement is essential. The necessary daily dose can vary from 5000 international units (IUs) to as many as 12000 IUs. I really like a vitamin D3 supplement known as Bio-D-Mulsion Forte by Biotics Research. I usually start patients on 2 drops by mouth, twice daily.

Careful monitoring of 25-OH vitamin D levels via regular blood work is essential. Based on results, the vitamin D3 dose might need to be adjusted.

Vitamin E

Vitamin E is an antioxidant with good evidence supporting its use. Studies have found a positive benefit in reducing cancer risk, including risk of lung and prostate cancer. (23) However, research on vitamin E has been conflicting. The SELECT trial, which looked at selenium and vitamin E supplementation on cancer risk, found that healthy men who supplemented with vitamin E had a significantly increased risk of prostate cancer. (24) Why the conflicting evidence?

The conflicting studies on vitamin E and cancer underscore the importance of taking the correct type of vitamin E. There are multiple forms of vitamin E, including dl-alpha tocopherol, d-alpha tocopherol, alpha-tocopherols, beta-tocopherols, gamma-tocopherols, and delta-tocopherols. The tocotrienol forms of vitamin E, namely the delta and gamma tocotrienols, are the correct form for anti-cancer purposes. Studies have shown that the tocotrienols, namely delta tocotrienol, affect multiple growth factors and signaling pathways in cancer cells. (25) These effects have been seen both in vitro and in vivo. The benefits of tocotrienols are not restricted to their anti-cancer activity; they also protect against cardiovascular disease, neurodegenerative disease, and immune system dysfunction. (26)

The SELECT trial used the alpha-tocopherol form of vitamin E. This form, which is one of the more common forms found in vitamin E supplements, depresses the levels of gamma and delta tocotrienols. By suppressing the tocotrienols—the anti-cancer forms of vitamin E—cancer risk increased. Of course, the headlines from the SELECT trial included none of these details, and instead warned of the "dangers" of vitamin E supplementation.

My preferred source of the tocotrienols is UNIQUE E Tocotrienols, a tocopherol-free formulation from A.C. Grace Company which contains delta and gamma tocotrienols. For cancer prevention, 1 capsule in the evening with food is the recommended dose. For cancer treatment purposes, I have patients take 2 capsules in the evening with food.

Zinc

Zinc is a trace mineral which is required by the body for proper cellular functioning. Several hundred enzymes in the body require zinc as a cofactor. However, zinc is also important for immune system health. Zinc deficiency has long been linked to immune system dysfunction; however, recent research has shown that zinc actually regulates the communication and signaling between immune system cells, and thus, the body's overall immune function. (27)

One important role of zinc as it relates to cancer formation and progression involves the tumor suppressor gene p53. We know that p53 regulates normal cell function, and virtually all cancers have a mutated p53 gene, allowing them to become immortal. Zinc is normally present on p53, and it has been shown that an abnormal amount (typically a deficiency) of zinc causes p53 to misfold. This greatly increases the risk of cancer development. (28) Interestingly, studies suggest that giving zinc might restore p53's normal function and thus inhibit tumor growth in cancer. (29)

An additional benefit of zinc is that it chelates copper. As we discussed previously, copper is frequently elevated in cancer patients and is required for the production of new blood vessels to feed tumors (angiogenesis). By helping to break down and eliminate copper, the angiogenesis process is negatively affected.

I recommend a chelated zinc, as this form tends to be better absorbed than non-chelated versions. I have one manufactured for my patients, and the typical dose is between 40-80 mg daily.

Note: I receive no financial compensation for recommending specific brands of supplements, nor do I have a financial stake in these companies. These are simply brands I recommend because they meet my high standards at the time of this writing. These recommendations are subject to change, as is the availability of these supplements sold by these specific companies. Often, supplement companies change ownership, leadership, or alter their manufacturing standards, which may in turn affect the quality of the supplements. It is important to research specific supplement companies and seek out the highest quality supplements available. Ideally, you should be under the care of an integrative oncologist who understands the nuances of supplements, has access to high quality supplements such as those mentioned here, and has the experience necessary to know how these supplements fit into a robust cancer treatment protocol.

(1) Fenton TR and Huang T. Systematic review of the association between dietary acid load, alkaline water, and cancer. BMJ Open 2016; 6: e010438.

(2) Damaghi M, Wojtkowiak JW, and Gillies RJ. pH sensing and regulation in cancer. Front Physiol 2013; 4: 370.

(3) Fais S, Venturi G, and Gatenby B. Microenvironmental acidosis in carcinogenesis and metastases: new strategies in prevention and therapy. Cancer Metastasis Rev 2014; 33(4): 1095-1108.

(4) Robey IF, Baggett BK, Kirkpatrick ND, et al. Bicarbonate increases tumor pH and inhibits spontaneous metastases. Cancer Res 2009; 69(6): 2260-8.

(5) Vetvicka V. B-glucans as Natural Biological Response Modifiers. Nova Science Publishers, New York, 2014.

(6) Fullerton, S A, et al. "Induction of Apoptosis in Human Prostatic Cancer Cells with Beta-Glucan (Maitake Mushroom Polysaccharide)." Molecular Urology., U.S. National Library of Medicine, 2000, www.ncbi.nlm.nih.gov/pubmed/10851301.

(7) Ina K, Kataoka T, and Ando T. The use of lentinan for treating gastric cancer. Anticancer Agents Med Chem 2013; 13: 681-8.

(8) Vetvicka V and Vetvickova J. Combination of glucan, resveratrol, and vitamin C demonstrates strong anti-tumor potential. Anticancer Res 2012; 32: 81-7.

(9) Epstein J, et al. Curcumin as a therapeutic agent: The evidence from in vitro, animal and human studies. Br J Nutrition 2010; 103(11): 1545–57.

(10) Khan N, Mukhtar H. Cancer and metastasis: Prevention and treatment by green tea. Cancer and Metastasis Reviews 2010; 29(3): 435–45.

(11) Warburg O. On the origin of cancer cells. Science 1956; 123: 3191.

(12) Warburg O. The metabolism of carcinoma cells. J Cancer Res 1925; 9(1): 148-63.

(13) Peskin BS. Report: "Scientific calculation of the optimum omega-6/-3 calculation." Houston: Pinnacle Press, 2008.

(14) Otto C, Hahlbrock T, Eich K, et al. Antiproliferative and anti metabolic effects behind the anticancer property of fermented wheat germ extract. BMC Complement Altern Med 2016; 16: 160.

(15) Langcake P, Pryce RJ. Production of resveratrol by vitis-vinifera and other members of vitaceae as a response to infection or injury. Physiological Plant Pathology 1976; 9: 77-86.

(16) Carter LG, D'Orazio JA, and Pearson KJ. Resveratrol and cancer: focus on in vivo evidence. Endocr Relat Cancer 2014; 21(3): R209-R225.

(17) Mukherjee S, Dudley JI, and Das DK. Dose-dependency of resveratrol in providing health benefits. Dose Response 2010; 8(4): 478-500.

(18) Willett WC, Polk BF, Morris JS, et al. Prediagnostic serum selenium and risk of cancer. Lancet 1983; 2(8342): 130-4.

(19) Lee EH, Myung SK, Jeon YJ, et al. Effects of selenium supplements on cancer prevention: meta-analysis of randomized controlled trials. Nutr Cancer 2011; 63(8): 1185-95.

(20) Bartolini D, Sancineto L, Fabro de Bern A, et al. Selenocompounds in cancer therapy: an overview. Adv Cancer Res 2017; 136: 259-302.

(21) Chen YC, Prabhu KS, and Mastro AM. Is selenium a potential treatment for cancer metastasis? Nutrients 2013; 5(4): 1149-68.

(22) Braumuller H, Wieder T, Brenner E, et al. T-helper-1-cell cytokines drive cancer into senescence. Nature 2013; 494(7437): 361-5.

(23) "How Vitamin E Helps Protect Against Cancer." The Physicians Committee, 20 July 2012, www.pcrm.org/health/cancer-resources/diet-cancer/nutrition/how-vitamin-e-helps-protect-against-cancer.

(24) Klein EA, Thompson IM Jr, Tangen CM, et al. Vitamin E and the risk of prostate cancer: the selenium and vitamin E cancer prevention trial (SELECT). JAMA 2011; 306(14): 1549-56.

(25) Kannappan R, Gupta SC, Kim JH, et al. Tocotrienols fight cancer by targeting multiple cell signaling pathways. Genes Nutr 2012; 7(1): 43-52.

(26) Meganathan P and Fu JY. Biological properties of tocotrienols: evidence in human studies. In J Mol Sci 2016; 17(11): 1682.

(27) Hojyo S and Fukada T. Roles of zinc signaling in the immune system. J Immunol Res 2016; 6762343.

(28) Loh SN. The missing zinc: p53 misfolding and cancer. Metallomics 2010; 2(7): 442-9.

(29) Puca R, Nardinocchi L, Porru M, et al. Restoring p53 active conformation by zinc increases the response of mutant p53 tumor cells to anticancer drugs. Cell Cycle 2011; 10(10): 1679-89.

CHAPTER 8

Mind–Body Medicine

"Do not conform to the pattern of this world, but be transformed by the renewing of your mind."
– Romans 12:2

What Is Mind-Body Medicine?

Upon introduction, mind-body medicine sounds somewhat esoteric. Indeed, I have many patients who come into my office who are somewhat skeptical when they first hear about it. Some patients are understandably hesitant about participating in anything which seems unfamiliar or at odds with their beliefs. The field, however, is anything but esoteric.

The mind-body medicine protocol we use in integrative oncology is derived from the burgeoning field of science that seeks to understand the close, intimate link between the brain and the rest of the body. For years, the mind, the brain, and the nervous system were viewed somewhat as a compartmentalized system within the body. In other words, there was the brain, and there was the rest of the body. What went on in the mind was not necessarily thought to influence the physical aspects of health and well-being.

Today, we know that there is an amazing network of connection between what goes on in the brain—including our thoughts, emotions, and even what we speak—and our body's physical health. For example, we now know that there is an enormous connection between thoughts and emotions and how our digestive system works. It is no coincidence that people who have anxiety are far more likely to have irritable bowel syndrome (IBS) and other digestive problems. We also know that there is a real connection between our thoughts and emotions and our immune system.

Really, this is not a terribly new idea. The notion that anxiety and stress can play a role, in heart attacks has been woven into our folksy wisdom for some time. The fact that we now have clear evidence that stress and anxiety influence factors such as blood pressure, that can then influence cardiac health, should serve as a prime example of how we know the mind influences our physical health in a real way.

The question becomes, do our thoughts and emotions—everything that goes on in our brains—influence the development of cancer, or how a patient responds to cancer treatment?

There is a good deal of published literature on the subject that affirms this. The field of psychoneuroimmunology is the study of the effect of the mind on health and resistance to disease. In the previous 30 years, there have been enormous strides in this field (one which was once considered outlandish in scientific circles). One of my professors at Georgetown University, Dr. Candace Pert, was one of the groundbreaking researchers in the field. Dr. Pert was among the first to demonstrate a clear connection between our emotions and the physical effects they could have on the rest our body. Even when I was a graduate student at Georgetown in the early 2000s, many of her contemporaries considered her, for lack of a better term, a nut. Fast forward to today, when she is recognized as a trailblazer, and her research is held in high regard by other scientists.

For our purposes, the conclusion among many prominent researchers in the field is that there are bio-behavioral pathways that can influence cancer development and progression. (1) In other words, what goes on in the brain plays a role in the development and progression of cancer.

A study published in 2013 sought to determine whether there is a link between the development of breast cancer and striking events in a woman's life. The study concluded that in women who had experienced some sort of significant, negative life event, the risk of breast cancer was increased by 1.5 times. Women who had experienced severely striking life events experienced a risk that was 2 times greater than women who reported no striking life events. The authors concluded that there was a positive correlation between striking life events and the development of breast cancer.(2)

These results are in keeping with the work of the German physician, Dr. Ryke Hamer, who was the first to posit the theory that certain life events contribute to the development of cancer. This is important, because this puts Dr. Hamer among the first to suggest that emotional trauma, or events that are experienced largely by the mind, can have a profound effect on our physical health.

Dr. Hamer's son was tragically and abruptly killed in an accident. Not long afterward, Dr. Hamer developed testicular cancer. He survived, but his experience led him to question whether there was a link between the emotional trauma he suffered following his son's death, and the development of his cancer.

Dr. Hamer went on to study thousands of cases of cancer, which included taking detailed histories of cancer patients. Ultimately, he concluded that striking life events and emotional traumas led directly to the development of certain cancers. Dr. Hamer was so convinced of what he had discovered, that by the end of his career, he was certain that he could predict not only what kind of cancer an individual would develop, but also the specific location within the body it would be located (within inches). All this simply by reviewing a patient's history!

Not surprisingly, Dr. Hamer's work was extremely controversial at the time, and still remains so. However, we are seeing affirmation of his theory in the scientific literature today. Simply, emotional trauma can and does influence the development of cancer.

A landmark study published about 20 years ago sought to compare two groups of breast cancer patients. The first group received the standard of care only; these women were treated with surgery, chemotherapy and radiation. The second group of women were given the standard of care as well, but in addition, they were placed in regular small group sessions. In these sessions, the women were taught stress reduction techniques, such as deep breathing and relaxation. These women were then taken through guided imagery, and instructed to imagine the cancer within their bodies dying and going away.

The results of the study were quite significant. The women in the second group had improved immune system function, less stress, and overall improved quality of life. (3)

Another study sought to determine whether mind-body medicine protocols could influence the physical pain experienced by cancer patients. Ultimately, the study found that there was a significant reduction in pain experienced in patients who received training in specific relaxation techniques, were taken through guided imagery, or received cognitive coping skills training. (4) Yet another study concluded that breast cancer patients who were provided relaxation, guided imagery, and biofeedback training experienced a reduction in anxiety and a boost in immune system function. (5)

These are only a few examples, but all point toward what much of the research coming out is telling us: there is a profound link between our mind and our body, and that link is evident both in cancer development and how the body responds to cancer treatment.

While mind-body medicine is a newer area of study, many of the larger, mainstream oncology centers are beginning to employ some of these strategies. This development speaks to how significant the research has become. In integrative oncology, however, we move beyond many of the basic therapy sessions employed by these larger treatment centers.

Instead, we strive to get to the heart of the emotional, spiritual, and mental side of cancer. We seek to address previous traumas, heal broken relationships, and mitigate the stressors inherent in both life and cancer treatment. By employing mind-body medicine, I believe we positively affect many of our patients' outcomes.

Addressing the Emotional and Spiritual Side of Cancer with Mind-Body Medicine

It is past time to address the fact that cancer is not just a physical disease, or a physical battle. Cancer has very real psychological, emotional, and spiritual sequelae, and those must be addressed as part of a comprehensive cancer treatment regimen. As Sir William Osler, considered the father of modern medicine, stated, "The good physician treats the disease; the great physician treats the patient who has the disease."

A cancer diagnosis often brings feelings of hopelessness, anxiety and despair. Often, a diagnosis blindsides otherwise healthy people, who—in an instant—are transported from their normal, healthy lives into the valley of the shadows of illness. The emotional, spiritual, and psychological implications of this are just as profound as the physical implications. Thus, it is critical that practitioners meet each patient in his or her journey, wherever that may be. Unfortunately, this is sorely lacking in conventional oncology.

Prior to starting medical school, I was a research intern at Harvard Medical School. My research project was on the doctor-patient relationship. I was intrigued by this sacred relationship, so much so that it was what drew me toward becoming a physician in the first place. However, what I found was that patients who have a strong relationship with their healthcare provider have better treatment outcomes. This relationship is built upon several key factors, including good communication, compassion, and ultimately, trust.

Once I became a practicing physician, I made it a point to emphasize the psychosocial aspects of a patient's life. This is especially true as it relates to a cancer diagnosis. In fact, a large section of my initial questionnaire for incoming patients revolves around details of their life before their cancer diagnosis. This includes questions about early childhood, whether a patient was abused mentally or physically, and if a patient has sustained any significant traumatic life events such as divorce or the loss of a loved one. These details are important; they speak to who a patient really is. After all, patients should be known as an individual, not merely as a diagnosis code or a case number.

As stated previously, we know that emotional trauma can set in motion a sequence of events inside the body which lead to cancer. (2) It is important to realize that science confirms that cancer is not just a disease of the biosphere; our mind, our emotions, our thoughts, and our spiritual health can—and almost always do—play a role in its incidence. Consequently, those same areas of our psyche can also be damaged by the diagnosis and treatment of the disease.

We can also use this to our advantage in our implementation of mind-body medicine. If we address some of the underlying emotional and spiritual factors that might have led to cancer's development, we can potentially affect outcomes in a positive way. Some of these tools, however, are not just beneficial for cancer patients, but for anyone trying to prevent cancer as well. Any comprehensive cancer prevention plan or cancer treatment protocol should implement some or all of the mind-body medicine strategies we will discuss.

Instilling Mindfulness

Because we know that our thoughts and our words have an effect on our minds (and ultimately our bodies), it is important for all people—not just cancer patients—to cultivate a sense of mindfulness. What this means is simply becoming more intentional about being present, or in the moment. Becoming more mindful means a heightened awareness about your thoughts, your mood, and your words.

A good example of the importance of mindfulness and how it can have consequences lies with food.

When was the last time you really sat down and savored the food you ate? Were you aware of the texture, the taste, and the smell? Many people cannot remember the last time they really sat down and enjoyed what they ate. So many of us are often in a rush, eating on the go, or throwing something pre-made into the microwave and scarfing it down as quickly as possible. Many of us reach for the first thing we see when we are hungry, never really thinking about what we are eating.

In many ways, we have seen the consequences of not being mindful about what we eat. In a country where a significant portion of the population is overweight or even obese, most people stand to benefit from being more conscious of what they are putting in their mouths. In fact, many books have been written about cultivating mindfulness with food, for the purposes of treating overeating or eating disorders.

Similar to how mindfulness with food may help control what we put into our bodies, mindfulness with our words and emotions can help us in controlling what we allow to come into our brain. Particularly, in the case of cancer patients, allowing your first panicked thoughts sweep over your mind and consume you is not a healthy way to deal with your diagnosis or your treatment.

This is not simply "positive thinking" for the sake of happiness or some sort of new age philosophy. Studies confirm that people who are positive do better with their treatments. One study of cancer patients concluded that mindfulness mediation resulted in a 65% reduction in mood disturbances and a 31% reduction in symptoms of stress. (6) These are very real outcomes, and if we are going to make a unilateral effort to fight cancer in the best way possible, addressing the power our thoughts and words possess must be taken into account.

Cultivating a sense of mindfulness paves the way for other strategies we use in our mind-body medicine protocol, such as mediation, prayer, and hypnotherapy.

Positive Confessions

There is an old saying that goes, "Whether you think you can or think you can't, you're right." This is likely not 100% accurate, but the essence of the saying is absolutely true; what we believe in our heart and confess with our mouth can and does have tremendous effect on the course of our life. Certainly, this is true as it relates to health, particularly when facing health challenges such as cancer.

There is no way around it, getting a diagnosis of cancer is a terrible and difficult thing to deal with. Understandably, it is easy for many cancer patients to lose hope, to become depressed, or to get lost in a sea of negativity. It is easy for cancer patients to fall into a repetitive line of thinking that says, "I am so sick, I feel terrible, and I am going to die."

Research, however, indicates that this is exactly the opposite of what we should be doing. There has been quite a bit of inquiry as to the effect our words have on our brains; much of this research indicates that what we say does influence our brains—and subsequently, our bodies—in a profound way. Margie Meacham, an expert on adult learning with a master's degree in the science of learning, says that, "…language doesn't operate simply at…the conscious level of the brain. We respond to words on a visceral, autonomic level, as well." In other words, the words we say and hear affect us on a level in the brain that controls our basic functions for living. Words affect us to our core. She goes on to say that, "…using positive words… can trigger the production of oxytocin, the neuro-chemical that helps trigger feelings such as well-being, affinity, and security…What we think about actually rewires our brains—for better or for worse." (7)

We can use this knowledge to our advantage with cancer treatment. One of the first things I do with my patients is give them a list of positive confessions to speak over themselves, and I ask them to recite them at least twice a day. I tell them to put them on their bathroom mirror, in their car, or on their phone, and to speak them out loud. Confessions such as, "I feel good," "I am healed," and "I am healthy" are simple and powerful. Saying these words aloud, coupled with maintaining a positive attitude, creates palpable, positive physical changes in the body. As Proverbs 18:21 tells us, "The tongue has the power of life and death, and those who love it will eat its fruit."

You can easily write your own daily confessions at home. I encourage you to not only focus your affirmations on your health, but also on other areas of your life including your family, your finances, etc. Any aspect of your life which is important to you warrants a place in your daily confessions. A logical extension of this is to combine it with your daily prayer and/or meditation time.

Hypnotherapy

Under 10% of our brain activity and thoughts are conscious. The remaining 90% of our brain activity is subconscious thought. Subconscious thoughts exert an enormous influence over our conscious thoughts, actions, and behaviors, as well as the functioning of our bodies. Since we know that our thoughts influence our physical health, it is important to recognize that our subconscious thoughts play a role in our health as well.

What happens, however, if those subconscious thoughts are tilted in a negative way?

Our subconsciousness can be influenced by the sum of our life events; particularly, negative events in our past can shape the way our subconscious thoughts flow in a negative way. In order to address these underlying problems in our subconscious, which inform many of our behaviors, we must access the subconscious somehow. This is where hypnotherapy plays a powerful role in mind-body medicine.

There are many myths, misunderstandings, and much misinformation about what hypnotherapy is, how it works, and what its utility is. Guided hypnosis is nothing like what you see in cartoons, or movies, or at "magic" shows, where a magician swings a pendulum and places someone in a trance, subsequently controlling their mind. Hypnosis is simply a deeper state of consciousness. With the help of a practitioner trained in hypnotherapy, patients can become more in tune with their subconscious way of thinking and gain access to their subconscious thoughts. This is done with the intent of addressing underlying problems therein. By addressing some of the problems in the subconscious that might have been instigated by life traumas many years prior, the aim is to confront these problems, and fix them. Subsequently, without the subconscious dominating the body in a negative way, we free the body to focus on positive endeavors, including healing from cancer.

Hypnotherapy is a well-studied mind-body medicine tool, used by many well-trained practitioners to help patients with a broad spectrum of health issues. People have used hypnotherapy to quit smoking, to fight addiction, and to overcome emotional trauma. To that end, its utility in fighting cancer has been the subject of serious scientific inquiry. Twenty-two clinical trials found that hypnotherapy is beneficial for cancer patients for the reduction of pain, anxiety, and stress associated with their disease. (8)

Many patients are often skeptical of hypnotherapy, largely because their view of it is based off of what they have seen in movies and television. In reality, hypnotherapy is a valuable tool in stress reduction, dealing with the challenges associated with cancer, and allowing the body to maximize its fighting abilities against the disease.

Daily Stress Reduction Techniques

If we look at the way our bodies are designed to deal with stress, it is clear that we are equipped to address acute stressors, such as life or death situations. This is where we hear the term "fight or flight;" whether you are running from a bear or fighting an enemy for your life, these are the situations your body's stress mechanisms are well-suited to handle. The body is remarkably adept at rallying in response to stress, up-regulating cortisol, adrenaline, and other hormones when they are needed until the stressor is removed. When the stressor is removed, the body is designed to return to normal.

The problem is that we live in an overstressed society, bombarded with negative news at every possible turn. We are more stressed than ever with regard to our family lives, finances, careers, and personal endeavors. We are also stressed about our health. None of these are the acute stressors we are optimally designed to deal with. Stress experienced in this way becomes chronic, not acute, and our body's stress mechanisms that were designed for sprinting are now forced to run a marathon, so to speak.

What happens is a resulting negative cascade of events. The adrenal glands (responsible for excreting the fight-or-flight hormone, adrenaline) become overworked. Cortisol goes up, which cannot be sustained, so it eventually goes down, creating stress on the adrenals. This subsequently affects your hormones, your immune system, your metabolism, your blood pressure, and even your blood sugar control, creating a situation in which the body is far from optimal in its functioning.

The easy thing to do is to remove the stressor that is the underlying cause of this cascade of events, but this is not always possible to do. Sure, we can mend certain relationships, or choose to live a less hectic lifestyle, or choose to eat healthier foods. Particularly, in the case of a cancer diagnosis, you cannot simply escape from, or remove, certain kinds of stressors. Ultimately, because we cannot eliminate stress altogether, our stressors must be dealt with or mitigated in a positive, healthy way. This is the role daily stress reduction techniques can play, not just in cancer treatment, but for anyone seeking to live a healthier life.

Deep Breathing Techniques

On the most basic level, deep breathing is one of the daily stress reduction techniques that we encourage in all of our patients.

Most people breathe too shallowly. For most, deep breathing may not become second nature or a completely regular habit, but we instruct all of our patients to take some time every day (or ideally, multiple times per day) to take deep, intentional, diaphragm-stretching breaths. It is important to breathe deeply so that not only the chest expands, but the stomach as well. Breathe in deeply for five seconds, hold for a few seconds, and then exhale the breath for five seconds. Doing this five or ten times can dramatically reduce levels of stress and anxiety. While deeply inhaling, imagine that you are breathing in peace, relaxation, and success. In contrast, when exhaling slowly, imagine eliminating stress, anxiety, and fear. This intentionality seems to help.

If you are feeling stressed or overwhelmed, or simply want to improve oxygenation to your body, this is an easy technique to employ anywhere.

Prayer & Meditation

From a Christian perspective, daily prayer time is a chance to clear your mind so that you can focus on God and listen to His voice. It is an important time to both cast your cares upon Him and also receive guidance. For many, particularly when facing cancer, prayer provides a time to focus on the central, most important pillar of your life: your relationship with the Holy Spirit.

We often think of prayer as a time to talk, communicating our thoughts, needs, wants, and requests to God. This is certainly an important aspect of prayer, as Philippians 4:6 tells us, "Be anxious about nothing, but in everything, by prayer and petition with thanksgiving, let your requests be made known to God." God certainly wants to hear from us! However, I feel strongly that we should also view prayer as a time to listen. As Romans 10:17 tells us, "Faith comes by hearing, and hearing by the Word of God." The Lord is regularly speaking to us, providing guidance, direction, and wisdom, but if we are not listening, we will not hear Him.

How is God speaking to you? Where is He leading you in terms of your cancer diagnosis and treatment? My prayer is that He is using the contents of this book to accomplish amazing things in your body and your life!

Meditation constitutes another form of quiet time, wherein meditators focus their thoughts and minds in a deep way. It is an excellent way to cultivate mindfulness, learn how to control your thoughts, and concentrate on what is important. There are many types of meditation—not necessarily just the spiritual or religious varieties—and readily available guides exist which teach one how to meditate. However you choose to do it, meditation should become a regular part of your routine.

Whether you spend time in prayer or in meditation, these are proven techniques for stress reduction, regardless of whether you are facing a diagnosis of cancer or not.

Emotional Freedom Technique

Emotional Freedom Technique, also known as EFT, was developed by Gary Craig, an engineer who also had an interest in psychology and personal improvement. EFT is a specific stress reduction method based on acupressure points that lie along the same meridians used in acupuncture. As a result, EFT has been called "psychological acupuncture." However, instead of using needles, EFT consists of tapping these pressure points on the face and body using the fingertips (but not so hard as to hurt). Tapping is performed while simultaneously thinking about specific problems or challenges (such as pain or specific life traumas) and verbally confessing positive affirmations to counteract these problems or challenges. Tapping on these pressure points introduces kinetic energy into these meridians. By introducing this kinetic energy whist speaking verbal affirmations over yourself, it serves to rid emotional blockages from your body's bioenergetic system.

Needless to say, many might be wary of this seemingly odd technique, but there is some good science backing up the use of EFT. The body can be thought of as an electromagnetic field, which is subject to both positive and negative influences. The negative disruptors of the body's electromagnetic field today are many, and are not limited to emotional stress. Radiation, microwaves, cellular phones, wireless internet routers, power lines, and even certain foods and chemical additives all serve as negative influences on the body's electromagnetic field and thus impact the body's normal functioning. EFT is one way to help bring the body's electromagnetic field back into balance. Emotional conflicts are neutralized at their source by restoring energy system balance.

Many practitioners use this technique to assist patients in dealing with pain, addiction, stress, and anxiety. EFT can also be used to help achieve positive goal setting and achievement. However, patients can easily learn it too, as a detailed knowledge of the Chinese meridian system is not required. Once patients learn the specific acupressure points, it is a technique they can easily employ on their own.

The EFT points are:

1. The karate chop point, located on the outside of the palm of the hands, halfway between the base of the pinky finger and the top of the wrist. This is the fleshy part you would use to perform a karate chop.
2. The top of the head point, located where the top of a baseball cap would be.
3. The eyebrow point, located over the inner eyebrow near the bridge of the nose.
4. The side of the eye point, just over the bone which runs along the outer portion of the eye.
5. The under the eye point, along the bone directly below the pupil.
6. The under the nose point, along the philtrum between the nose and upper lip.

7. The chin point, between the lower lip and upper portion of the chin.

8. The collarbone point, at the center U-shaped portion at the top of the sternum.

9. The underarm point, about four inches below the armpit along the side of the breast.

The basics of EFT are as follows:

1. Identify a problem to work on. Examples include anxiety about a cancer diagnosis, worry about undergoing cancer treatment, and fear of dying.

2. Determine how much this problem, and its resulting anxiety or discomfort, bothers you on a scale of 0-10 (0 = no distress, and 10= highest level of discomfort).

3. Choose an affirmation statement. If the problem you identified was, "I have anxiety about my cancer diagnosis," your affirmation statement might be "Even though I have this anxiety about my cancer diagnosis, I deeply and completely accept myself."

4. Perform the setup. Using the index finger, middle finger, and ring finger simultaneously, begin tapping on the karate chop point (point 1) while stating your affirmation statement aloud three times.

5. After completing step 4, identify a brief phrase to remind yourself of the problem you want to work on. Using our example from above, "my cancer anxiety" would be a good reminder phrase.

6. Tap the stress relief points (points 2-9) one by one, stating your reminder phrase ("my cancer anxiety").

7. Rate your anxiety or stress again, using the 0-10 scale above. If the problem is no longer bothering you, you can stop. However, if there is still some discomfort present, repeat the setup (step 4) and go through the steps again. This time, you will revise your affirmation statement to reflect that you are making progress. For

example, you might say, "Even though I still have some anxiety about my cancer diagnosis, I deeply and completely accept myself."

8. Continue this procedure as many times as desired.

As you can see, EFT is safe, non-invasive, and easy to apply. I encourage you to give it a try. It might seem odd at first, but it works!

Other Forms of Daily Stress Reduction

Some methods of stress reduction are right in front of us, yet often we miss them. Just because they are common, however, does not mean they do not impart some benefit, nor does it mean we should exclude them from our regimen. Truly, there are simple ways of reducing stress every day—and methods that have been shown to play a significant role in stress reduction and improved health. These are strategies in which we should all commit to engaging.

The first of these is laughter. When was the last time you truly laughed? Laughter has been shown to reduce stress and boost immunity (9). Understandably, people who are diagnosed with cancer typically do not spend a lot of time laughing. Simply watching a movie that makes you laugh or spending time with people who do the same should be an important and regular part of your life. The more stressed you are, the greater laughter's importance should become.

Human touch is another action that has been shown to reduce stress. (10) Simply getting and receiving a hug from someone can boost levels of oxytocin and endorphins. This is important for cancer patients as well as their loved ones. Physical touch can be a small but important aspect of stress relief and maintaining good spirits throughout trying times.

Listening to soothing music is also another easy way to reduce stress levels. (11) Music can be relaxing and enjoyable, and constitutes a simple way to find time to relax and relieve stress.

All of these forms of daily stress reduction do not have to be followed, but incorporating at least some of these into your daily regimen is a healthy way to mitigate stress on a daily basis. If we are going to fight cancer—either preventatively, or as part of a treatment protocol—stress reduction through a variety of methods must become an important component of our overall strategy.

Healing Relationships

Part of addressing the emotional side of cancer involves healing relationships that have been damaged. In my personal experience, I find that the majority of the patients who come into my practice have a history of significantly broken relationships, whether from a traumatic childhood, a past divorce, death of a loved one, or an estranged child. According to researchers such as Dr. Hamer and others, it certainly seems that stressors such as these contribute to the development of cancer.

For many people, relationship stress has been present for years. This is, in part, why the mind-body medicine component of a treatment protocol is so important. Addressing the broken relationships in one's life is a vital component of the healing process. I have seen the mending of relationships positively affect cancer treatment outcomes. When relationships are strengthened, a burden is lifted from the body, and healing physical ailments (in this case, cancer) can be prioritized.

In addition to resolving negative or stressful relationships, it is also essential to build and maintain strong, positive, and healthy relationships. Evidence suggests that patients with supportive relationships have better treatment outcomes. Nurturing your support system is a powerful way to positively influence your treatment outcome.

Goals and Maintaining Quality of Life

For someone who has been diagnosed with cancer, it is vital to set goals for yourself. For many, the goal should (and can) be complete removal of cancer from the body and a return to full, vibrant health. For others, especially those with very advanced cancer, the goal might be to stabilize cancer so that it becomes a chronic disease which can be managed, allowing for a good quality of life. Goal setting for the short, medium, and long-term is very important.

Regardless of your stage and type of cancer, setting small, measurable goals is essential. As my late mother, Dr. Susan Stegall, taught me from a young age, "Break the process down into doable parts." Intentional goal-setting not only makes a daunting task more manageable, but it also allows us to experience small victories early on. This serves as positive reinforcement, while consciously and subconsciously instructing the mind and body to get accustomed to winning. Each goal accomplished represents one step closer to healing.

Whether you are a stage I patient, a stage IV patient, or somewhere in between, it is important to prioritize quality of life. Many of the treatments we use in integrative oncology are geared toward effectively treating cancer while also maintaining a good quality of life. I believe that this should not only be measured with regard to physical health, but also mental, spiritual, and emotional health. Addressing health in this holistic fashion is the only way to achieve true healing.

●━━━━━━━●

(1) Green McDonald P, O'Connell M, Lutgendorf SK. Psychoneuroimmunology and cancer: a decade of discovery, paradigm shifts, and methodological innovations. Brain Behav Immun 2013; 30: S1-9.

(2) Lin Y, Wang C, Zhong Y, et al. Striking life events associated with primary breast cancer susceptibility in women: a meta-analysis study. J Exp Clin Cancer Res 2013; (32)1: 53.

(3) Richardson MA, Post-White J, Grimm EA, et al. Coping, life attitudes, and immune responses to imagery and group support

after breast cancer treatment. Altern Ther Health Med 1997; 3(5): 62-70.

(4) Arathuzik D. Effects of cognitive-behavioral strategies on pain in cancer patients. Cancer Nurs 1994; 17(3): 207-14.

(5) Gruber BL, Hersh SP, Hall NRS, et al. Immunological responses of breast cancer patients to behavioral interventions. Biofeedback Self-Regul 1993; 18(1): 1–22.

(6) Speca M, Carlson LE, Goodey E, et al. A randomized, wait-list controlled clinical trial: the effect of a mindfulness meditation-based stress reduction program on mood and symptoms of stress in cancer outpatients. Psychosom Med 2000; 62(5): 613-22.

(7) Meacham, Margie. "How Words Affect Our Brains." Association for Talent Development, 2017, www.td.org/insights/how-words-affect-our-brains.

(8) Boehm K, Horneber M. "Hypnotherapy." Hypnotherapy / Mind-Body Interventions / CAM-Cancer, 29 Apr. 2016, cam-cancer.org/The-Summaries/Mind-body-interventions/ Hypnotherapy.

(9) Bennett MP, Zeller JM, Rosenberg L, et al. The effect of mirthful laughter on stress and natural killer cell activity. Altern Ther Health Med 2003; 9(2): 38–45.

(10) Dworkin-McDaniel, Norine. "Touching Makes You Healthier." CNN, Cable News Network, 5 Jan. 2011, www.cnn.com/2011/ HEALTH/01/05/touching.makes.you.healthier.health/index. html.

(11) Thoma MV, La Marca R, Bronnimann R, et al. The effect of music on the human stress response. PLoS One 2013; 8(8): e70156.

CHAPTER 9

Cancer Myths and Magical Thinking

"True knowledge exists in knowing that you know nothing."
— *Socrates*

The Age of Information and Misinformation

Never before in history has there existed such an abundance of information in virtually every field imaginable. Since the Enlightenment and the birth of the scientific method, our knowledge of science has increased on an exponential slope. The field of medicine, like all other fields of scientific inquiry, has progressed beyond our ancestors' wildest dreams.

In the last 50 years, breakthroughs in medical research and advancements in technology have greatly increased our knowledge of the human body. The capabilities medical science now has in terms of imaging, testing, diagnostics, surgery, and drug therapy would have likely seemed like science fiction, even for people in the middle of the last century. As far as medicine is concerned, it is a fascinating time to be alive.

Like many other fields, the advent of the internet has had many implications on health and medicine. Notably, the internet has put much of the information that comprises the canon of literature on health and medicine at the fingertips of not just people in the medical field, but also for all people. This is a wonderfully empowering tool, yet it is not without its own set of side effects.

The Pros and Cons of the Internet

Most of the patients who discover me and my practice are well-educated and have done quite a bit of research on their own. Not surprisingly, much of this research occurs through the internet. Many of these patients have doubts about conventional oncology, and many have a great deal of hope that some of the things they have researched online can truly help them. Many are simply relieved to find an oncologist who is open-minded.

It is important to remember, though, that open-mindedness without a healthy level of skepticism is likely just as bad as a purely closed-minded outlook on oncology, medicine, or really any field of inquiry. Many patients are disappointed to find out that I often disagree with some of the ideas they bring to the table. Often, I have to tell patients that some of the therapies they read about on the internet have no evidence to support their use and are likely a waste of time, if not downright harmful.

This highlights one of the negative impacts the internet has had on cancer care: there is simply a wealth of misinformation, particularly with regard to which alternative treatments might be beneficial for cancer. Particularly with the advent of social media, the internet has become an open forum, with little or no vetting of information that gets disseminated. Anyone with or without qualifications can post virtually whatever they want on the internet, even on seemingly legitimate websites or through avenues that appear reputable.

Understandably, cancer is a hot topic, and any information regarding potentially beneficial cancer treatments (particularly treatments outside of the standard of care) typically spreads like wildfire through the internet, garnering quite a bit of traffic for any site that posts such information.

Unfortunately, many readers who are understandably hopeful for a natural cancer cure are left believing that they just read legitimate news.

Another negative impact the internet has had, particularly on cancer patients, is a feeling of overwhelm as a result of the volume of information, whether it is good information or not. Notwithstanding the fact that most lay people do not have the scientific literacy to accurately assess the implications of most scientific studies, even sifting through legitimate, published, scientific studies on the varieties of alternative treatments that might be beneficial for cancer care can create a sort of "paralysis by analysis." Even preliminary research is often overwhelming for patients and their families, and it can be difficult to discern what information is good information and then process that information into any sort of useful action.

The fact that there is both a wealth of good information available along with so much misinformation, however, serves to underscore the crucial role of the integrative oncologist. One of my roles is to help patients navigate the ocean of information and misinformation available to them so that we can both decide what treatment options—both conventional and alternative—are likely to be beneficial in their fight against cancer. This is what a doctor-patient relationship should look like.

As we discussed previously, what should exist between doctor and patient is a respectful exchange of information, not the paternalistic paradigm to which many have grown accustomed. Sadly, many patients today feel powerless when it comes to having a say in their own treatment, and sense that they are being looked down upon by their doctor. Patients need—and deserve—the latitude to ask questions about whether certain treatments could be beneficial, and to provide input as to the treatments they desire. However, the physician still needs—and has earned—the ability to advise patients regarding a reasonable course of action. Some patients want to take patient-focused care and turn it into patient-dictated care, which is just as damaging as paternalistic doctors are to the doctor-patient relationship. A true balance of power between doctor and patient is what is needed, with a net result which is only positive.

Many patients come to me after having done extensive independent research. Most are eager to try alternative therapies, and often, they will bring information or studies they have found on the internet into my office. Often, many of my patients will want to incorporate therapies they have read about on the internet into their treatment regimen. What I do is openly and honestly discuss the research they have found. Is what they have found based on a scientific study? If so, was it a good study? Was it a lab study done on cells, or was it done on animals? Or, was it studied in humans? Was the study done over a short or long period of time? Did it involve a small or large number of patients? Did the study have a control group, or was it a case control study? Was the study biased in any way? All of these questions matter a great deal.

These criteria for assessing scientific studies can provide us with vital information about the level of evidence for whether a certain treatment might have benefits for a particular case. Often, I will assign a "level of evidence" grade ranging from A through F. An A-level study is typically done in humans over a longer period of time, and constitutes a high level of evidence for safety and efficacy. In contrast, D- or F-level studies constitute lower levels of evidence which tell us nothing about whether or not they work in humans. I generally try to dissuade patients from trying therapies with such low level of evidence, especially as a sole means of treatment. Some of these therapies might have some promise, but we simply do not have the level of evidence currently that would suggest that their use has any benefit. Sometimes, however, we will incorporate some of these therapies into a regimen, just not to the exclusion of treatments for which we have good evidence.

Typically, most patients are not bringing in large, double blind, placebo-controlled studies conducted by large pharmaceutical companies or via large grants from the government. While those types of studies certainly constitute the highest level of evidence, they also run the risk of being inherently biased. In addition, these studies typically do not involve alternative therapies. However, we do not exclude alternative treatments simply because many of the studies conducted on them are less than ideal. It simply means that we have more research to do. In the meantime, if the evidence we have indicates that a therapy might be helpful and will not harm a patient, why would we not try it?

This is one of the primary roles of the integrative oncologist. Medical training renders physicians capable of properly interpreting information within the volumes of published medical research available, and then using those results to come up with real-world applications. Unfortunately, most physicians today possess neither the intellectual curiosity nor the willingness to consider therapies outside the scope of conventional medicine. In contrast, integrative oncologists tend to possess a rare combination of clinical experience and intellectual curiosity, thus creating a clear path to treating cancer with both conventional and alternative medicine.

What I have described is perhaps the most beneficial impact of the internet. The internet is helping us to collectively shed the paternalistic view long-held in medicine, where the doctor is always right and the patient has no say in his or her treatment. The information available online can be very empowering to cancer patients, as it should be. In conjunction with an integrative oncologist trained to help analyze both the good and misleading information that is available, the internet can prove to be a powerful tool in the hands of cancer patients.

7 Common Myths about Cancer

With the widespread dissemination of misinformation via the internet, numerous myths about cancer exist and continue to be perpetuated. Often, these center around conspiracy theories related to "Big Pharma," the government, or some other shadow entity that wishes to withhold knowledge of a cure for financial reasons, or even out of pure malevolence.

Interestingly, one of the side effects of the internet has been that these sorts of beliefs are not relegated to the fringe anymore. Many educated and otherwise "normal" people often have this paradigm as part of their worldview, in varying degrees. Many are suspicious of government and the pharmaceutical industry, and this has led to their interest in so-called "alternative" medicine. With the greed and lying we have seen within industry and government, it is difficult to blame people for being suspicious. Some suspicion is likely a good thing. Unfortunately, this paradigm can make people vulnerable to believing things that might not be supported by fact, particularly when it comes to alternative cancer treatment methods.

Myths about cancer are not relegated to the alternative or natural side of the debate. There are myths about cancer that are perpetuated on the conventional side of cancer care, too. Many of the things you will hear from a conventional oncologist simply do not stack up against what we know to be true about cancer.

We in medicine need to do away with the idea that we sit in an ivory tower or that we are necessarily right about everything. This view is shortsighted and is not always beneficial for our patients. In fact, we should be reminded of what Dave Sackett, MD, considered the father of evidence-based medicine, had to say: "Half of what you will learn in medical school will be shown to be dead wrong or out of date within five years of your medical school graduation." Needless to say, it is time for conventional medicine to realize that there are treatments outside of the conventional scope, with solid evidence to back their use, and that some of the current cancer paradigms are outdated.

Myth #1: Cancer Is a Genetic Disease

Sometimes, cancer is the result of mutated genes that we inherit from our parents, but even our most aggressive estimates only put the percentage of cancers that are purely genetic at between 6-8%. (1) This leaves the overwhelming majority of cancers to be attributed to another cause. Furthermore, recent study into the blossoming field of epigenetics calls into question whether genes, or mutated genes, are really to blame in the instance of cancer—or if the environment to which we expose those genes plays the majority role. Research into cancer, however, has largely centered around the genetic component, leading many oncologists to believe that cancer is purely genetic in nature. What that research has largely neglected, though, is what caused the mutation in those genes to begin with. In essence, we have focused, and are still focusing, most of our research and drug development efforts on the roughly 5% of cancer that has a genetic cause, and neglecting the 95% which does not.

You will recall that cancer has a very primitive way of producing energy in comparison to a healthy cell. Healthy cells go through a long metabolic process that results in the production of 32 to 36 units of ATP, the energy currency of cells. Cancer only goes through the first portion of that process, known as glycolysis, to create ATP. Glycolysis is the process by which cells metabolize sugar in the form of glucose for energy, meaning cancer is very reliant on a steady source of sugar to create energy. This difference between a healthy cell and a malignant cell is a key hallmark of cancer. This distinction is so important that it has led some forward-thinking researchers to the conclusion that cancer is more of a metabolic disease than a genetic disease.

When we talk about cancer as a metabolic disease, we are referring to cellular metabolism, or the way a cell produces energy. Dr. Thomas Seyfried is one of the pioneers in researching the metabolic component of cancer. In his book, *Cancer as a Metabolic Disease*, he references a deep study that helps highlight some of the flaws in the idea that cancer is purely genetic. Instead, the study strongly emphasized the metabolic nature of the disease.

In the study, researchers took the nucleus (the part of the cell where all the genetic material is held) of a cancer cell and implanted it into an otherwise healthy cell. All of the other cellular structures, such as the cell membrane, the cytoplasm, and the mitochondria, were healthy. Interestingly, and to the surprise of most researchers, that cell did not become cancerous. Conversely, the researchers took the nucleus of a healthy cell and implanted it into a cancerous cell. That cell went on to replicate in the same way a cancer cell would. (2) This leads us to the conclusion that the other structures in the cell, most notably those which are responsible for energy production, are the key players in the process of cancer formation. Thus, cancer is not genetically driven, it is metabolically driven.

We know that if our cells are under constant bombardment by being bathed in a toxic environment, they become worn down far more quickly than they otherwise would. As cells become worn out, they do not produce energy as well. These multiple "hits" on a healthy cell are what I believe trigger the metabolic changes that lead to damaged DNA, and ultimately to cancer. Our cells can sustain a certain amount of hits, but when our toxic bucket is full, it overflows; our cells simply cannot indefinitely withstand toxic bombardment. Ultimately, our cells mutate in order to stay alive. On a very basic level, this can be thought of as cellular aging.

Certainly, genes and genetics play a role in cancer. That role, however, is likely quite overstated. Calling cancer a genetic disease is a misnomer at this point. On the other hand, when we view cancer as a metabolic disease, we open ourselves up to a wider variety of effective treatments against the disease. This is especially true since the research into cancer as a genetic disease has largely been a failure with regard to developing curative treatments.

Finally, we must acknowledge the small percentage of cancers which have been deemed "genetic." Based on the aforementioned studies, it is very likely that the cancer genetics which were passed down from parent to child originally resulted from metabolic derangements. The principles we use for fighting cancer in these cases still very much apply, with the only difference being that the metabolic damage has existed for a longer period of time.

Myth #2: Biopsies and Surgeries Should Be Avoided Because They Spread Cancer

Typically, a biopsy of a tumor involves a needle that penetrates the tumor to collect cells. The data gathered from a biopsy can establish a cancer diagnosis and provide potentially life-saving information on the type of cancer in question. In fact, it is a critical step in the diagnostic process. Many people who suspect that they have cancer are often afraid to get a biopsy, or outright refuse them, for fear that the biopsy itself will spread the cancer.

There are two kinds of needle biopsies. A fine needle aspiration biopsy (FNAB) uses a needle that has a very small hollow core, allowing the collection of very few cells. The second kind of biopsy involves a needle with a larger hollow core, known as a core sampling, and provides an increased sampling of cells from a tumor. In both cases, there are accounts within the medical literature that indicate a process known as tract seeding can take place, in which cancerous cells left behind in the path of the needle enter the blood stream and travel to remote organs and grow into new tumors. These cases, however, are exceptionally rare. So rare, that in cases of prostate cancer biopsies, the likelihood of tract seeding is thought to be much, much less than 0.001%, by the most aggressive estimates. (3)

Regardless, in 2008, an article published on the website Medical News Today came with the headline, *Prostate Biopsy Spreads Prostate Cancer Cells*. Though the article was quickly refuted by a prominent urologist (4), it is headlines like these that often spread very quickly via the internet, inciting fear in patients. Even after they are refuted, these types of articles continue to be shared and spread throughout the internet.

While tract seeding is an extremely rare, albeit documented, side effect of biopsies, particularly in more aggressive cancers, the benefits of biopsies overwhelmingly outweigh the risks, even in cases of cancer that are ostensibly most at risk for tract seeding. In 2014, the Mayo Clinic published a study that followed over 2,000 pancreatic cancer patients over the course of 11 years. What the study found was that the group of patients who had a needle biopsy had noticeably better outcomes than those who did not. The study did not find any evidence of tract seeding in patients who had a needle biopsy. (5)

Ultimately, biopsies are an important diagnostic tool that improve cancer outcomes, and much of the fear surrounding them is stoked by misinformation on the internet. While tract seeding can occur, it is so rare as to be considered clinically irrelevant by most physicians—including me.

Similarly, many patients refuse surgery for fear that the surgery will spread cancer. One theory as to how this belief started is because people will naturally feel worse for a period of time after surgery. This has nothing to do with surgery spreading cancer, but is instead the body's normal response to an invasive procedure such as surgery.

However, a recent study in mice found that there is a risk of cancer spread after breast cancer surgery. (6) Surgery does create an inflammatory environment, and this environment—and the resulting wound healing which must occur—does increase the risk of cancer spread. Interestingly, the study found that the mice who were given nonsteroidal anti-inflammatory drugs (NSAIDs) mitigated the increased risk of cancer spread.

It is important to remember that surgery is often the best first line of defense against cancer, assuming that the tumor is accessible via surgery. In some instances, when a tumor is so large that surgery is not an option, we may choose to try to shrink it with chemotherapy and then operate. Chemotherapy given in this manner is known as neoadjuvant chemotherapy, as the focus is on first shrinking the tumor to create a better environment for surgery. In the absence of such a situation, it is almost always a good idea to get a tumor removed as quickly as possible.

When patients tell me that they are afraid that surgery spreads cancer, I kindly remind them that leaving a cancerous tumor inside the body spreads cancer at an exponentially higher rate!

Proper use of NSAIDs such as ibuprofen or celexocib in the post-op setting is something I recommend, not only for decreasing metastatic risk from surgery, but also for reduction in inflammation and pain. If you are a surgical candidate, get that tumor out so that the source of cancer is removed! Doing so makes our job of addressing the systemic burden of cancer much easier.

Myth #3: What You Eat Does Not Matter

Nutritional information with regard to cancer is abundant, but much of it is conflicting, misleading, and likely wrong. Perhaps the biggest myth, though, when it comes to cancer and nutrition is that it simply does not matter what you eat. This is a myth promoted by conventional oncology, despite their claims that they practice evidence-based medicine.

We know that diet can play a valuable role in cancer treatment, and is surely useful in its prevention as well. We know that foods like processed meats and alcoholic beverages are on the list of Group 1 carcinogens. Nitrates and nitrites (often found in processed foods), glyphosate (a common pesticide used in conventionally grown crops), and fried foods are among the Group 2A carcinogens. (7) Conversely, it is also published that lifestyle factors, such as diet, play a role in the incidence of cancer, and that by simply changing some these factors, it is estimated that over half of cancers could be prevented. (8) It is well documented that certain vegetables, fruits, and foods high in fiber reduce the risk of developing cancer. (9)

Many patients who visit my clinic have already seen a conventional oncologist. In that setting, nutrition is usually a topic initiated by patients, not doctors. When these patients ask their oncologist if they should be eating a specific diet, they are almost always told, "It doesn't matter what you eat." At most, their oncologist tells them not to lose too much weight for fear that doing so could worsen cachexia—the wasting syndrome resulting in weight loss, fatigue, weakness, and muscle atrophy. Cachexia can be fatal, so I understand their concern.

Wasting is responsible for nearly 30% of deaths related to cancer. Once you see a patient die from cachexia, you never forget it. However, according to research, appropriate nutritional intervention can stabilize or reverse weight loss in as many as 50-88% of cases. (10)

Simply put, it matters what you eat. Nutrition plays a valuable and significant role in treating cancer, as well as reducing some of the side effects of the treatments which are sometimes employed. As we have already discussed, our key nutritional principles are centered around a plant-based diet, focusing on minimally-processed organic foods, methionine restriction, and intermittent fasting.

Myth #4: Cancer Is Easily Curable Using Natural Methods Only

A large part of why people turn to natural remedies is that they have experienced some of the terrible side effects of conventional cancer treatments. Side effects such as hair loss, nausea, vomiting, diarrhea, skin rashes, weakness, fatigue, and weight loss are just some of the ones we commonly see. Most of us have watched as loved ones died not from cancer necessarily, but from the side effects of the treatments. Other patients have seen conventional cancer treatments fail to work as promised, and seek out alternative treatments with the hope that these methods can offer better outcome.

The idea that cancer can be easily cured using natural methods is largely fueled by information available online. The problem is, most of the information people get online exclusively promoting natural cancer treatments has little to no scientific backing. Many of the claims are unsubstantiated at best, and some are simply wrong. Much of the information is anecdotal. There are many people who claim to have treated their cancer naturally with good outcomes. Admittedly, this does happen. There are case histories in which patients who were sent home to die with stage 4 cancer changed their diet and took supplements and miraculously went into remission. There are also cases of people who did nothing to treat their cancer who spontaneously went into remission. Estimates as to the frequency of these occurrences are approximately 1 in 100,000 cases. (11)

It is extremely important to remember that these accounts of miraculous natural cancer cures are the exception, and by no means the rule. Overwhelmingly, evidence suggests that patients who attempt to treat their cancer with only natural remedies, or patients who do nothing at all, experience very poor results. A study published by Yale University sought to examine treatment outcomes from the exclusive use of alternative therapies, and found that it results in a lower survival rate. (12) The study found that patients who chose to forgo conventional treatment, and instead incorporated only alternative treatments, were as much as 5 times more likely to be dead in five years compared to those who used conventional cancer treatments. Unfortunately, my personal experience as a physician largely backs up what these researchers found. However, it is important to note that this study did not examine specific alternative therapies, which means that those in the study were likely using a wide range of alternative treatments.

For some, this might be a hard reality to face. After all, we *want* to believe that there are consistently reliable natural cancer cures out there. The idea that we can use natural treatments which are both effective and safe, with little to no side effects, to exclusively treat cancer and obtain never-before-seen results sounds amazing. My hope is that we will get there one day, but unfortunately, we are not there yet.

Relying on natural therapies alone to treat cancer is akin to purchasing a lottery ticket; you might win, but it is unlikely. For every lottery winner you see on television, there are thousands—maybe even millions—who purchased a ticket and lost. It is the same way with those who try to treat their cancer with nutrition and supplementation alone.

This is not to say that alternative or natural therapies do not have evidence supporting their use or efficacy. While not all of these treatments are useful or effective, some absolutely are, and I believe that we should employ those modalities whenever possible, but in conjunction with more proven and established therapies. My personal belief is that there are likely undiscovered cures in nature, but at this point we remain unsure of what they are, how they work, and how to implement them clinically. Until those treatments are discovered and fully understood, it is shortsighted and irresponsible to try to treat cancer with natural therapies exclusively, or to expect good results if you choose to do so.

It is true that the side effects of conventional cancer treatments can constitute a decline in quality of life, but rejecting conventional treatment altogether—simply because it is not perfect or ideal—constitutes a drastic and inappropriate response to these concerns. The answer is not to throw out the treatments for which we have strong evidence, while relying exclusively on treatments with little or no evidence. The risks to your life and health nearly always outweigh the benefits of choosing to fully reject chemotherapy and other conventional treatments in favor of natural treatments. It is important to remember that there are volumes of evidence supporting the use of chemotherapy, surgery, and radiation, which is why they are still used. How those therapies are used can have a huge bearing on their efficacy and the incidence of side effects. This is why integrative oncology makes use of these conventional therapies, often in very innovative ways, and combines them with evidence-based natural and alternative therapies. This is a best-of-both-worlds approach.

Myth #5: Cures Are Being Withheld from You by Big Pharma

Conspiracy theories existed long before the internet, but never before have like-minded people been able to find a community as easily as they do online. The internet has served to concentrate people that believe a wide array of conspiracies. The ability of these people to so easily reinforce each other's thinking has only allowed those ideas to grow and subsequently disseminate.

The psychology of conspiracy theories is interesting in its own right. Often, it is easier for some people to cling to the idea that there is someone, or a group of people, in the shadows "pulling the strings" that cause bad things to happen, than it is to accept that we live in a fallen world with complex problems that are difficult to solve. As a huge industry dealing in serious life-or-death matters, the medical industry has been one of the primary targets for conspiracy theorists.

Cancer is obviously an easy target for conspiracy theorists. Certainly—in the minds of conspiracy theorists—there is a simple cure available, but it has been withheld by malevolent forces, such as "Big Pharma," actors within the government, or a shadowy cabal of world leaders. The motivation for such evil behavior is typically money; conventional cancer treatments are big business, particularly if they are patented. This is coupled with the misleading statements about doctors getting kickbacks from the pharmaceutical industry, or that surgeons only want to operate, etc.

Never mind that this assumes the worst about an enormous swath of people, the myth that there would be no money in a cure for cancer is simply false. One estimate in 2006 placed the value of a cure for cancer at over $50 trillion. (13) Many conspiracy theorists' answer to this is that if a cure is natural, it cannot be patented, therefore, drug companies will not release said cure, because they, exclusively, could not profit from it. Again, if this were the case, why has not one drug company executive started a supplement company selling a natural cure for cancer? For people who are exclusively profit-minded, not doing this would simply be shortsighted!

Ultimately, treating cancer is not profitable simply because of the pharmaceutical industry, but because cancer is so prevalent. This also makes a cure incredibly valuable; so valuable, in fact, that if it were ever found, it would be rushed to market through whatever avenue would be most efficient.

Conspiracy theorists have always existed, but they have largely been relegated to the fringe in terms of their influence over the majority of people's ideas. What is interesting about how the internet has changed our collective perspective, particularly regarding cancer, is that the demographic of people who ascribe to these sorts of ideas has changed. There is a growing segment of the population, many of whom are well-educated and hold college degrees, that believe these sorts of conspiracy theories.

Some of this is fueled by sensationalism. Anytime a study implicates any natural therapy in treating cancer, it spreads like wildfire through blogs, social media, and other online avenues. People see these studies on the efficacy of vitamins, herbs, or supplements and think, why is this not used in place of chemotherapy? Sadly, for many, this only reinforces the idea that these safe, simple, and all-natural cures are being withheld from them by the powers that be.

I am here to tell you, as a physician whose primary aim is to see my patients get well, who does not have stock in a drug or supplement company, and who desperately wants a natural cure for cancer: there are no known cures for cancer. The search for a cure motivates me and keeps me awake at night, and I can assure you that it has not been found yet. I will be the first to let you know when it has!

Myth #6: If Something Kills Cancer in a Petri Dish, It Will Kill Cancer in the Body

We regularly see attention-grabbing headlines online, particularly on social media, of natural substances killing cancer cells. A recent one which made its rounds online was, "Frankincense kills cancer better than chemotherapy!" Since we are regularly bombarded with these types of headlines, it makes sense that many people wonder why these natural treatments are not being used in place of more toxic treatments like chemotherapy.

It is important to remember that many of the websites that post these types of sensational headlines are often trying to direct as much traffic to their sites as possible. Many of these sites are, in essence, paid based on the traffic they receive since they sell advertising space. Some of these websites are also generating traffic in order to sell their own products. Many well-intentioned readers succumb to this research as being applicable to themselves or a loved one with cancer.

There is a progression that all research into potentially effective treatment compounds must follow. The first step in this process is studying a compound in a laboratory setting outside the body, also known as *in vitro*. A compound is placed in a petri dish with cancer cells, and the effects are observed. This is known as a cell line study. Many kinds of vitamins, minerals, plant extracts, and other compounds have been studied for a variety of anti-cancer properties in this setting, and many have been found to be effective in killing cancer in some regard. Sounds great, right?

Before we get too excited about substances killing cancer cells *in vitro*, it is important to point out that bleach kills cancer cells very well in a petri dish as well. Of course, we do not want to swallow or inject bleach thinking that it would confer any type of health benefit, because we know that bleach is toxic. Yet, when lab studies come out on essential oils such as frankincense, some people assume that means that using frankincense in the body amounts to a cure, because they do not equate frankincense with toxicity. As we have discussed in earlier chapters, it is very important to remember that any substance, natural or synthetic, which has a potential effect in the body also has the potential to have toxicity within the body. This is why additional studies beyond cell line studies are so important, because we must examine the true effectiveness of a substance as well as the proper and safe dosing of that substance.

Furthermore, there is published evidence indicating that many cell line studies are deeply flawed. Cell lines are cell cultures developed from single cancer cells. As cancer cells are essentially immortal (having lost the apoptosis mechanism healthy cells have, which limits their lifespan), they can be grown for extended periods in laboratory settings so that they can be studied. These cell lines are provided to researchers by only a few companies worldwide. Unfortunately, there is evidence that much of the research conducted on cancer cell lines has been done on cultures that have been contaminated, or incorrectly designated. This casts doubt on much of the research done for specific cancers and the compounds which might be effective against them. (14)

Effectiveness *in vitro* tells us very little about what will happen *in vivo*, or inside the human body. Whether a substance will be effective, as well as safe, in the body for treatment purposes requires a great deal of additional research. There are a wide variety of factors that laboratory studies do not address, including:
  – How will a compound react in the body if swallowed?
  – How will a compound react in the body if injected?
  – What are the side effects of this compound?
  – What is the toxicity level?
  – Is there a safe dose which is still effective?
  – Is it metabolized before it reaches its site of action?

If a compound does show promise in the lab, the next step typically involves studies wherein a promising compound is administered to animals. Many of the compounds that might have shown promise in a laboratory setting might not behave the same way in an animal study, and some wind up having no efficacy at all. However, those compounds which do show effectiveness in animals typically warrant further study.

The final step is taking compounds which have shown promise in a laboratory setting and in animal studies and testing their safety and efficacy in humans—*in vivo*. This constitutes a huge leap from studying a compound in a laboratory. Often, years of research (and lots of funding) are needed before a compound can be adequately studied in humans.

Sometimes, we find substances which are effective, and they go on to become drugs. Often, compounds simply do not work in humans, even if they are effective in animal studies. Make no mistake, the human body is an incredibly complex physiological and biochemical environment. In fact, a potential cancer treatment which shows effectiveness in animal studies has a very low likelihood of having that success replicated in human studies. In fact, only about 8% of animal studies end up working in humans. (15)

An important caveat here is that many substances—especially natural substances—which have shown benefit in cell line and animal studies have not undergone rigorous studies in humans. Because extensive human studies involve so much funding, and because most studies are funded by entities such as pharmaceutical companies which stand to profit from patenting the substance under study, it becomes obvious why non-patentable natural substances are not the subject of long-term human studies. This puts us between a rock and a hard place with regard to many integrative and alternative cancer treatments; we see promise in these treatments, and want to see more rigorous studies on them, but there has not been—and likely never will be—such studies, because there is no one to pay for them. So at best, we are left with smaller human studies. Although these studies are not ideal, they do provide some evidence we can use.

Returning to our earlier example of frankincense, it might be a wonderful cancer treatment. In fact, I am not against its use, and it seems to be safe when used properly and might even provide an anti-cancer benefit. So we might employ it as part of an integrative cancer treatment protocol, but not instead of more proven treatments.

Myth #7: Alkaline Diets Cure Cancer

As we have discussed, there is much misinformation available on the internet which can spread very quickly. This is particularly true as it relates to nutrition advice. One of the most recent examples of this sort of dietary fad is the alkaline diet.

The basic tenets of the alkaline diet state that certain foods can change the pH of the body. The alkaline diet claims to shift the pH of the body away from the acidic end of the spectrum—which according to this theory, promotes disease—to the more alkaline end of the pH spectrum, which ostensibly promotes health. The alkaline diet encourages foods that would promote alkalinity, such as fruits, vegetables, nuts, and beans, and shuns foods thought to promote acidity, such as meat, dairy, eggs, grains, and alcohol. Interestingly, sugar is thought to be neutral, making the alkaline diet one of the only cancer diets not vehemently opposed to sugar—something that has unequivocally been linked to a variety of diseases, including cancer. This, alone, should be cause for suspicion.

Among the claims made by proponents of the alkaline diet is that it cannot only prevent cancer, but cure it, as well. Not all proponents of the alkaline diet believe this necessarily, and this is not to say that the alkaline diet does not confer some health benefits. Most of these benefits, however, come from simply eating healthier varieties of foods and excluding many unhealthy ones.

Any claims, however, about diet somehow shifting the pH of the body are rooted in some misunderstandings about biochemistry and how the human body functions. As discussed previously, the kidneys regulate the body's pH within a very narrow range. In the presence of healthy kidneys, eating an alkaline diet will not alter the pH inside the body. Drinking alkaline water in particular might actually do more harm than good; alkaline water is simply neutralized when it meets stomach acid, forcing the stomach and the kidneys to work harder. Stomach acid, too, is beneficial. It assists in digesting food and acts as a frontline of defense against invading pathogens. Neutralizing that acid, or making that part of the body more alkaline, is not a good idea. The alkaline diet typically calls for strict monitoring of the body using pH strips to test the saliva and/or urine. When eating a more alkaline diet, both urine and saliva will soon become more alkaline as well. Don't fall for the trap of believing that this reflects a more alkaline body. Rather, this is evidence of the body doing its job, as the body will rid itself of excess alkalinity (or acidity, depending on the situation) to maintain the blood pH around 7.4.

The importance of pH in cancer is real, but it has been generalized into what is a myth. Unfortunately, eating an alkaline diet will not do much to address the pH properties of cancer that are worth addressing; recent studies have concluded that alkaline diets and alkaline water are not supported by research and that their promotion to treat or prevent cancer is unjustified. (16) Anyone claiming otherwise likely misunderstands the mechanism behind the pH of cancer cells, or how it can be clinically used against the disease. However, focusing on a plant-based, organic, and minimally processed diet, and ensuring that the body's digestion, elimination, and detoxification are working optimally, is precisely what the body needs in order to best fight cancer. And you do not have to use pH strips to measure your saliva or urine!

———•———•———

(1) Garber JE, Offit K. Hereditary cancer predisposition syndromes. J Clin Oncol 2005; 23(2): 276-92.

(2) Seyfried TN. Cancer as a mitochondrial metabolic disease. Front Cell Dev Biol 2015; 3: 43.

(3) Sperling D. The Truth About Biopsy. Sperling Prostate Center, sperlingprostatecenter.com/truth-biopsy-track-seeding/. Accessed 17 Aug 2017.

(4)   Whittington R. Prostate Biopsy Spreads Cancer Cells? OncoLink, www.oncolink.org/frequently-asked-questions/cancers/prostate/prostate-biopsy-spreads-cancer-cells. Accessed 17 Aug 2017.

(5)   Punsky K. Mayo Researchers Find Cancer Biopsies Do Not Promote Cancer Spread. Mayo Clinic, Mayo Foundation for Medical Education and Research, newsnetwork.mayoclinic.org/discussion/mayo-researchers-find-cancer-biopsies-do-not-promote-cancer-spread/. Accessed 17 Aug. 2017.

(6)   Krall JA, Reinhardt F, Mercury OA, et al. The systemic response to surgery triggers the outgrowth of distant immune-controlled tumors in mouse models of dormancy. Sci Transl Med 2018; 10(436): eaan3464.

(7)   "Known and Probable Human Carcinogens." American Cancer Society, www.cancer.org/cancer/cancer-causes/general-info/known-and-probable-human-carcinogens.html. Accessed 17 Aug. 2017.

(8)   Song M, Giovannucci E. Preventable incidence and mortality of carcinoma associated with lifestyle factors among white adults in the United States. JAMA Oncol 2016; 2(9): 1154-61.

(9)   "How healthy eating prevents cancer." Cancer Research UK, 7 Apr 2017, www.cancerresearchuk.org/about-cancer/causes-of-cancer/diet-and-cancer/how-healthy-eating-prevents-cancer. Accessed 17 Aug 2017.

(10)   Food and Drug Administration: U.S. Department of Health and Human Services. 2004. Innovation or Stagnation: Challenge and Opportunity on the Critical Path to New Medical Products.

(11)   Fauvet J, Campagne J, Chavy A, et al. Cures, Regressions, and Spontaneous Remissions of Cancer. La Revue du Practicien 1960; 10: 2349-84.

(12)   Johnson SB, Park HS, Gross CP, et al. Use of alternative medicine for cancer and its impact on survival. J Natl Cancer Inst 2018; 110(1): 121-24.

(13) Murphy KM, Topel RH. The value of health and longevity. J Pol Econ 2006; 114(5): 871-904.

(14) Lacroix M. Persistent use of "false" cell lines. Int J Cancer 2008; 122(1): 1-4.

(15) Collective, The Tincture. "Nutrition and Cancer: Where do we go from here? – Tincture." Tincture, Tincture, 4 Mar. 2016, tincture.io/nutrition-and-cancer-where-do-we-go-from-here-7f93632e0464. Accessed 21 Aug. 2017.

(16) Fenton TR, Huang T. Systematic review of the association between dietary acid load, alkaline water, and cancer. BMJ Open 2016; 6: e010438.

CHAPTER 10

Cancer Prevention—8 Tips From an Integrative Oncologist

"An ounce of prevention is worth a pound of cure."
– Benjamin Franklin

Understandably, most people try to avoid thinking about diseases such as cancer as much as possible. Unfortunately, many are forced to think about cancer far more than they ever wished, due to a diagnosis in a loved one or even themselves. Because cancer is going to affect all of us in some form or fashion, we should all spend some time thinking about ways to prevent it from ever occurring. According to research, as much as 40% of cancer could be prevented, solely by making some simple lifestyle changes. (1)

Prevention is likely the biggest missing piece in the conventional discussion on cancer. Typically, most people would never speak to an oncologist unless they have already been diagnosed with cancer. At that point, a discussion on prevention is not the most pressing matter. Oncologists work in treating cancer, not preventing it, and to that end, we often have little advice when it comes to reducing cancer risk. The role of discussing cancer prevention should lie with a family doctor, internist, or gynecologist, but aside from basic screening such as prostate exams, mammograms, and Pap smears, such advice is sorely lacking. Most conversations about cancer prevention between doctor and patient are extremely limited, especially in comparison to other major health issues in our society such as heart disease.

As far as mainstream advice, there is little extra in regards to what you can do to prevent cancer. We are told to eat a healthy diet, not to smoke, avoid alcohol, and to exercise. These are fine lifestyle tips, but given the rate at which cancer is becoming the biggest killer of Americans, this advice is insufficient at best. Even with all of the advancements conventional oncology has made, and despite utilizing every tool in the integrative oncologist's tool chest, cancer will continue to be a complex disease to treat for the foreseeable future. If we are to win the war on cancer, it must start with a serious discussion about prevention.

We also must work to remove the outdated notion that cancer is a purely genetic disease. Many people are relegated to a life of worry, thinking that because they have a relative who had cancer, they are doomed to receive a cancer diagnosis, as well. On the other hand, people who think they are immune to the disease because they have no cancer in their families need to realize that they are essentially at just as much at risk as those who do have a family history of cancer. Ultimately, regardless of your genes, the choices you make and the environment to which you are exposed have an enormous amount of influence over the health you do—or do not—enjoy.

The Toxic Bucket

As discussed in the previous chapter, the myth that cancer is a purely genetic disease has likely set us back in terms of our discussion on cancer prevention, because it has removed the focus on what I believe the main underlying causes of cancer actually are. When we look at the genetic changes we see in cancer, they are almost always the result of a wide variety of environmental exposures which have damaged the metabolism, or energy mechanisms, of the cell.

As we now know, much of the early work of Dr. Otto Warburg, along with the current work of Dr. Thomas Seyfried and others, points toward cancer being a metabolic disease as opposed to a disease of genetics. Work in the relatively new field of epigenetics—or, the role environmental factors play in the expression of genes—also points toward cancer being a metabolic disease. The question then becomes, what are the forces at work disrupting the metabolic processes within our cells?

It is helpful to think of our cells as a bucket. Each "hit" that they incur from a wide variety of negative environmental exposures accumulates, like a hose slowly dripping into a bucket. Our cells can tolerate a certain amount of those accumulated hits, but eventually they become old and worn-out prematurely; the bucket fills up. In a way, we can think of this as cellular aging. The cells do not manufacture energy or perform their vital functions the way they were intended.

Eventually, the bucket fills to the top with accumulated cellular insults, and it overflows. Our cells can only withstand so much. This is when we see cells become cancerous. Our cells mutate in order to survive the toxic environment in which they are constantly bathed.

Our discussion on cancer prevention must focus on the way we prevent our toxic bucket from overflowing. In other words, how do we create an environment in our bodies which is conducive to preventing cancer from developing? This question has an ever-evolving list of answers, but there are certainly some things we can confidently recommend, based on science as well as common sense. My tips in this section are not only important for those hoping to prevent cancer; they are also essential for those fighting cancer.

Tip 1: Avoid Carcinogenic Environmental Exposures

Often, people equate carcinogenic environmental exposure to working in or living near a factory, power plant, or landfill. While these exposures are certainly likely to increase cancer risk, many other toxic sources do as well—and their prevalence is not isolated to one of the aforementioned locales.

Since the dawn of industrialization, and the subsequent explosion of new chemical compounds available on the market since World War II, we have routinely—and often unknowingly—been exposing ourselves to dangerous and toxic chemicals. In some instances, we have learned the hard way that many of the products we have invented have deadly side effects, such as asbestos. Today, however, we take many elements of our industrialized society for granted. As a result, we rarely stop to think about what we are necessarily exposing ourselves to on a day-to-day basis. From the air we breathe, to the cosmetics we apply, to the cleaning agents we use, we expose ourselves regularly to chemicals which are causing us harm.

At this point in civilization, it is impossible to completely avoid exposure to toxic chemicals, but we should not ignore these exposures simply because we cannot fully prevent them. Certainly, not everything we expose ourselves to in our everyday environment is going to cause cancer. At the same time, we cannot—and should not—rely solely on regulatory bodies to tell us what is safe and what is not. The truth of the matter is that many of the chemicals which we are regularly exposed to are not tested for long-term safety. Because of this uncertainty, the best course of action is to be as aware as possible of our surroundings, and mitigate our exposures to potentially carcinogenic agents as best as we can. Remember, our cells can thankfully withstand a certain number of hits without our toxic bucket overflowing.

To some extent, minimizing our exposure to carcinogenic environments requires more awareness and a certain amount of lifestyle change. It is frightening to think about how toxic our environments have become, and reducing our toxic exposures is an essential factor in preventing cancer.

What We Breathe

When we talk about respiratory exposures causing cancer, the general assumption is that we are referring to tobacco smoke. The advice not to smoke is perhaps the most often heard advice when it comes to cancer prevention, and rightfully so. Smoking is still the leading cause of cancer. This is a well published fact, yet people continue to smoke. Quitting smoking is one of the best preventative measures one can take for not only reducing risk of lung cancer, but a variety of other cancers, as well.

A discussion about smoking would not be complete without also covering passive smoking, also known as secondhand smoke. Soon after the link between smoking and various cancers was proven, researchers began to uncover increased cancer rates in those who were exposed to secondhand smoke. Not surprisingly, the greater the extent of exposure to secondhand smoke, the higher the risk of cancer. While most municipalities have greatly reduced the number of indoor spaces where smoking is allowed, smoking indoors is still legal in many places. Avoid such environments as much as possible.

It is important to emphasize that other kinds of smoke, including marijuana as well as e-cigarettes, do not constitute safe alternatives. Anytime you inhale combusted material, you are breathing carcinogenic particulate, which increases the risk for cancer. Even cigar smoking, where one does not typically inhale, increases risk for developing multiple cancers.

Smoking, however, is not the only thing we must be concerned about when it comes to what we breathe. Every time you take a breath, air from the environment around you fills your lungs, where oxygen enters the bloodstream through tiny blood vessels. Oxygen is not the only component of air to enter the body, though. To the contrary, any contaminants or pollutants in the air will also enter the bloodstream, requiring the body to address—and hopefully eliminate—all of them.

Indoor Spaces

Indoor spaces are particularly vulnerable to being contaminated with aerosolized chemical contaminates. Many building materials, such as new paint or carpet often "off-gas," which is frequently accompanied by chemical smell. Furnishings such as mattresses and sofas are full of harmful chemicals. Other materials, such as the leather and vinyl used in new cars, also off-gas into the confined space of a car. While many people enjoy the "new car" smell, these fumes represent known toxins. In fact, some of them have been linked to cancer. (2)

Another problem not often discussed is the presence of mold in indoor spaces. Mold and mildew are known to cause a variety of health problems, such as asthma and allergies, but certain molds also produce carcinogenic poisons, known as mycotoxins. Mycotoxins can become aerosolized and inhaled in contaminated spaces. (3)

Radon gas is also something which people should test for in their homes. Radon is an odorless, tasteless, and invisible gas that is the result of decaying, naturally-occurring uranium in the soil. It is able to seep through cracks in foundations and contaminate indoor air. Radon has been shown to elevate cancer risks, particularly in smokers, but there is evidence for elevated cancer risk in anyone who is exposed. (4)

There is evidence that indoor pollutants play a role in causing cancer. Many indoor pollutants can be avoided, but some cannot. It is important to remember that when we are talking about cancer risk, we are talking about the aggregate effect of all "hits" on our cells—our toxic bucket overflowing. Mitigate these indoor pollutants whenever possible.

Some ways you can mitigate indoor pollutants are:
- Do not smoke, or allow smoking of any kind in your home or car. Avoid establishments that allow indoor smoking.
- Keep your home well-ventilated, and open windows when possible.
- Use green building materials, such as eco-friendly carpeting, underlays, and paint.

- Be careful when purchasing new furniture, as many varieties frequently contain harmful chemicals which are off-gassed into the air.
- Do not allow your home or work space be contaminated with mold; clean any visible mold.
- If you suspect mold colonization in areas not visible, test the air quality in your home.
- Have your home tested for radon gas. If levels are high, take proper mitigation steps.

Outdoor Pollutants

Outdoor air pollutants come in a wide variety of forms, from motor vehicle exhaust to factory waste. Outdoor air pollution can contain diesel exhaust, dust, solvents, and aerosolized heavy metals.

Air pollution is an unavoidable part of our modern society. Unfortunately, there is evidence that it can be quite carcinogenic. In 2013, a panel organized by the International Agency for Research on Cancer (IARC) concluded that there is enough evidence proving that air pollution causes cancer in humans. Specifically, a component of air pollution called PM 2.5 (particulate matter, or dust-like particles, less that 2.5 millionths of a meter across) could be labeled as likely causing cancer. Specifically, this type of air pollution is linked to lung cancer and bladder cancer. (5, 6)

The risk of developing lung cancer as a result of air pollution is thought to be small, and regulatory officials in developed countries have gone to great lengths to reduce levels of air pollution over the last forty years. People living in developing countries are likely at a greater risk for problems associated with air pollution. Regardless of where you live, there are a few things you can do to mitigate this risk:
- Avoid being outside as much as possible on days when there is an air alert.

- Avoid breathing exhaust from cars, buses or other combustion engines. This is much easier in rural and suburban areas than in urban areas.
- Avoid living or working close to any coal or fossil fuel burning facilities.

Exposures via Skin

What our skin comes into contact with every day constitutes another method of exposure to potentially harmful compounds. What is striking is the number of chemicals we are exposed to every day, often without thinking about it. Consider a day in the life:

Most people get up out of their dyed sheets that were cleaned with chemical-laden detergent to get ready for work, or to get their kids ready for school. Some might shave with shaving cream, or brush their teeth with toothpaste, then use mouthwash. Often, one will step into a warm shower; the water in the shower is clean by standards in other parts of the world, but it does contain chlorine, fluoride, and other dissolved minerals which likely increase cancer risk. Then comes soap, shampoo, and conditioners. After getting out of the shower, many people apply deodorant or antiperspirant. Often, a variety of hair-styling products are used. For many women, makeup is applied. A clean set of clothes— perhaps cleaned at the dry cleaners—are put on, perhaps a bit of some sort of fragrance is applied, and you are out the door.

This is all before leaving your home, or coming into contact with any other environmental exposures. Thinking exclusively about the ingredients in each of those cosmetics mentioned above, you begin to realize the long list of *hundreds* of chemicals people expose themselves to on a daily basis, just via the skin. Some of these have been tested extensively for long-term safety; unfortunately, most have not. To be honest, we simply do not know what the long-term effects of exposure to certain chemicals in our cosmetics are. Chances are, they are not beneficial, and many are likely harmful.

Some of them, however, we do know are linked to cancer. Ingredients such as phthalates, parabens, and talc are among the ingredients regularly listed on the labels of beauty products, and all have evidence suggesting a role in cancer development. (7,8,9)

Unfortunately, that awareness regarding what we expose our skin to must extend beyond the cosmetics we use. There is evidence that even materials like mattresses and furniture that use flame retardant materials elevate cancer risk. (10) The chemicals in these types of furniture can absorb through the skin on contact, or release fumes which are then inhaled. Fortunately, steps have been taken in recent years by regulatory bodies to remove some of the volatile organic compounds from furniture and other consumer products. (11) Of course, much more needs to be done.

There is evidence that other exposures via the skin also elevate cancer risk. Studies suggest that the chemical known as perchloroethylene or tetrachloroethylene (also known as PERC) used in dry cleaning elevates cancer risk. (12) Even the water we bathe and swim in might elevate our risk for cancer. When chlorine reacts with organic compounds, there are byproducts created, including trihalomethane (THM) and haloacetic acid (HAA), and these have been shown to cause cancer in laboratory studies. (13)

This seems like an overwhelming amount of information to be concerned about, does it not? Sadly, the truth is that we are floating in toxic soup virtually all the time. Although it is scary when first learning that many of the consumer products we buy are likely harmful, it is also empowering to know that these risks exist so that steps can be taken to minimize the potential damage. Again, what we are concerned about is the cumulative effect of all these hits to our cells. Certainly, in the case of cancer, we want to diminish the overall risk our environment poses when it comes to damaging our cells.

While it seems that industry is not always in our corner when it comes to protecting consumers, there are advocacy groups which strive to evaluate consumer products for safety, particularly when it comes to cancer risk. One of those is the Environmental Working Group (EWG). This non-profit group evaluates thousands of consumer products for safety. Interestingly, out of over 70,000 cosmetic products they have reviewed at the time of this writing, less than 1,000 have received an EWG certified approval for safety. (14)

In today's world, it is virtually impossible to completely avoid environmental exposures that elevate cancer risk. However, there are some recommendations I can confidently make:

- Research the ingredients in your cosmetics; opt for more natural ingredients when possible.
- Avoid chemicals used in dry cleaning.
- Research household items like cleaners, detergents, and soaps; opt for greener and more natural varieties.
- Avoid indoor and/or chlorinated swimming pools; opt for salt-water pools when possible.
- Install whole house water filters in your home if possible.
- Avoid furniture or mattresses that use flame retardant materials.

Tip 2: Maintain a Healthy Weight

It is important to have a definition of what being overweight and/or obese is. Our best method for determining whether or not a person is overweight is likely still body mass index, or BMI. There are a number of problems with BMI calculations, the most notable being that they do not take into account bone density or muscle mass. Still, it is a good guide for the majority of people to assess whether they are in the generally accepted proper weight range.

BMI is calculated by dividing your weight (in kilograms) by your height (in meters) squared. The formula looks like this: kg/m2. If you weigh 90 kg (approximately 200 lbs) and you are about 2 meters tall (about 6 feet), your BMI is 22.5. A BMI under 18.5 is considered underweight. Between 18.5 and 24.9 is considered normal. If you are between 25-29.9, you are considered overweight; anything over 30 is considered obese. Ideally, one should aim to be in the normal BMI range, between 18.5 and 24.9. Most people in the United States, however, do not fall into this range.

It is no secret that there is an obesity epidemic in the United States. Between 1988-1994, 56% of adults were considered overweight. However, between 2011-2014, it was estimated that 70% of adults in the United States were considered overweight, while 36.5% were considered obese. Similarly, overweight and obesity rates in children have also risen dramatically. Between 1988-1994, the obesity rate for children ages 2-19 was approximately 10%; by 2011-2014, as many as 17% of children in this age group were considered obese. (15)

There are a variety of factors thought to play a role in the obesity epidemic, including sedentary lifestyle, poor diet, and environmental exposures. There are many known health risks associated with obesity, including heart disease, diabetes, osteoporosis, and others. Most people do not realize, however, that being overweight or obese significantly increases your risks for a wide variety of cancers, including endometrial cancer, esophageal cancer, stomach cancer, liver cancer, kidney cancer, pancreatic cancer, colorectal cancer, gallbladder cancer, breast cancer, and ovarian cancer, to name a few. (15)

There are a variety of mechanisms thought to drive the increased risk of cancer due to obesity. People who are overweight have an increase in estrogen, due to fat cells' production of estrogen, which plays a role in hormone-driven cancers such as breast, ovarian, and prostate cancers. In addition, estrogen promotes inflammation, which certainly supports the theory that cancer is a metabolic (or inflammatory) disease. People who are overweight tend to produce more insulin and insulin-like growth factor (IGF-1) than those people who are within normal weight ranges. You will recall that cancer cells have a much higher number of insulin and sugar receptors on their cell surface, meaning that for people who are overweight, the heightened amount of insulin and IGF will work to stimulate cancer cells.

Ultimately, maintaining a healthy weight is one of the most critical factors for preventing cancer from developing in the first place.

Tip 3: Do Not Get Type II Diabetes

Type II diabetes is a disease in which your body is either resistant to insulin, or your body does not produce enough insulin to maintain proper blood glucose levels. Insulin is a hormone made by the pancreas that regulates the way cells process glucose, or sugar, into energy. More than 27 million people have diabetes in the United States, but as many as 86 million are thought to be pre-diabetic, meaning they have high blood glucose, but not quite high enough to be considered diabetic. (16)

There are a variety of risks associated with diabetes, including heart disease, nerve damage, kidney damage and damage to the eyes, but developing type II diabetes also puts one at a higher risk for developing cancer. Type II diabetes is thought to double the risk of liver, pancreatic, and endometrial cancers, but the risk is also elevated for colorectal cancer, breast cancer, and bladder cancer. (17)

The reasons for this increased risk are clear. In diabetics, the pancreas is forced to excrete more and more insulin to maintain proper blood glucose levels as cells become more and more resistant to insulin. We know that cancer is stimulated by insulin and glucose—two things found in much higher levels of diabetics. Type II diabetes is largely a lifestyle disease as well; we see the same risk factors that elevate one's risk of cancer also elevate the risk of developing diabetes, such as sedentary lifestyle, poor diet, and higher levels of inflammation. These attributes might also account for the increase in cancer risk associated with diabetes. This upward trend in insulin production, however, is also the case in pre-diabetics, meaning that the 86 million people or so in the United States are not immune to the heightened cancer risks associated with diabetes.

Fortunately, diabetes and pre-diabetes are both largely preventable by changing some lifestyle factors. Maintaining a healthy weight, eating a diet low in sugar and refined carbohydrates, and regular exercise all play a role in the prevention of type II diabetes, and subsequently in preventing cancer as well.

Tip 4: Do Not Lower Your Cholesterol Too Much

Cholesterol is a much-maligned nutrient. We have all heard the public service announcements about the dangers of high cholesterol, and seen the ad campaigns promoting the newest cholesterol lowering drugs. Most Americans believe that cholesterol is bad, and that having it as low as possible is ideal. However, what many people do not know is that cholesterol is a necessary building block for cells, is involved in the manufacturing of hormones such as vitamin D, is needed for proper immune system function, and even plays a role in digesting food. Your body manufactures all the cholesterol necessary for bodily functions, but some is available from foods like eggs, meat, and dairy.

Most of us only think of heart disease when we think about maintaining healthy cholesterol levels. We naturally have cholesterol in our blood, but excessive levels of cholesterol are thought to lead to blockage in the arteries; excess cholesterol collects in the arteries, forming plaques that block blood flow to the heart, which is the primary cause of heart disease. For years now, cardiologists have been putting patients on cholesterol-lowering drugs with the aim of preventing heart disease. This was also the thrust behind low-fat diets, which eliminated a lot of cholesterol-rich foods from the diet.

Despite all of the dietary recommendations made, and the millions of people on cholesterol-lowering medications, heart disease has remained the leading cause of death in the United States. Interestingly, however, in recent years, research has pointed toward inflammation as much more important underlying cause of heart disease than high cholesterol. Inflammation, it appears, is what causes cholesterol in the blood to oxidize, forming the plaques that block blood flow. As with many other diseases, including cancer, inflammation lies at the root of the problem.

This is not to say that high cholesterol is a good thing, necessarily. The reality is that our definition of what constitutes high cholesterol is probably incorrect, and is probably slightly different for each person based on age, lifestyle, family history, and existing health issues.

Regarding the relationship between cholesterol and cancer, think twice before lowering your cholesterol too much. A 2012 study found a correlation between people with low LDL cholesterol (who had never taken cholesterol medication) and an increased risk of developing cancer. (18) This study was not particularly conclusive, but it is important to note that a relationship exists between low LDL cholesterol (thought to be the "bad" kind of cholesterol) and risk for developing cancer later in life. Whether the risk is correlative or causal remains to be seen. Regardless, it highlights another positive role cholesterol likely plays in the body.

Tip 5: Avoid Certain Viruses

When most people think of viruses, typically, they think of catching a stomach bug, the flu, or at the very worst, HIV. Needless to say, viruses are not typically associated with cancer.

A virus, however, was one of the first discovered causes of cancer. In 1911, Peyton Rous would discover what would be called the Rous sarcoma virus, a virus that causes cancer in chickens. (19) Since then, there have been a variety of viruses shown to elevate the risk of cancer in humans. While getting any one of these viruses does not guarantee one will get cancer by any means, the elevated risk associated with contracting these viruses is simply another reason to avoid becoming infected with them.

Epstein-Barr Virus (EBV)

Epstein-Barr is responsible for causing mononucleosis ("mono"), also known as the kissing disease. Most people in the United States are infected with EBV before the end of their teen years. It can be contracted through kissing, sneezing, coughing, or sharing eating utensils. Once you have been infected with the virus, it remains in your body indefinitely. (20)

EBV has been linked to nasopharyngeal cancer, certain lymphomas, and some cases of stomach cancer, but given its prevalence, cancer cases associated with it are very rare. EBV does not cause serious health problems in most people, and very few people infected with the virus will ever develop cancer as a result.

Hepatitis B & C Viruses (HBV and HCV)

HBV and HCV both can infect the liver, causing chronic, viral hepatitis. Both of these viruses increase the risk of liver cancer. Less than half of liver cancers in the United States are associated with HBV or HCV, but that rate is higher in other parts of the world. (20) Both HBV and HCV can be contracted via shared needles, or by having unprotected sex with an infected person. Both viruses can be spread through childbirth. Blood transfusions can spread these viruses, but this is extremely rare in the United States, since all blood used for transfusions is tested for these and other viruses.

There is a vaccine for HBV, but not for HCV. For both viruses, treatments are available to sometimes cure (in the case of HCV) or mitigate damage to the liver (in the case of HBV). Treating the viruses lowers the risk of developing cancer as a result of infection.

Avoiding the associated risky behaviors is the best way to prevent infection of both HBV and HCV, and thus reduce cancer risk.

Human Herpes Virus 8 (HHV-8)

HHV-8 is a virus spread through unprotected sex and possibly through saliva and blood. Fewer than 10% of people in the United States have this virus. (20) Also known as the Kaposi sarcoma-associated herpes virus (KSHV), HHV-8 is found in virtually all Kaposi sarcoma (KS) tumors. KS often appears as reddish-purple or blue-brown tumor just below the skin. It is rare and very slow-growing. HHV-8 might also be linked to certain types of lymphoma.

Most people with HHV-8 never go on to develop KS. However, it is thought that in addition to being infected with the virus, other factors like a weakened immune system can lead to the development of KS in people with the virus.

Human Papilloma Viruses (HPV)

Human papilloma viruses, or HPVs, are comprised of over 150 different types of viruses; among those, at least 12 are thought to cause cancer. HPVs are spread through contact (touching) and over 40 are spread through sexual activity.

HPV infections are very common. In fact, most sexually active people are infected with one or more types of these viruses at least once in their lifetime. Because these viruses are so common, the development of cancers as a result of HPV infection is relatively rare. In other words, the majority of people infected with these viruses do not develop cancer. (20) However, some HPVs are the primary causes of cervical cancer, the second most common cancer in women. HPV has also been linked to cancers of the penis, anus, vagina, vulva, mouth, and throat. One of the reasons we are hearing more about HPV, particularly in regards to cancer, is that there has been an increase in the number of head and neck cancers associated with HPV. These cancers are likely the result of oral sex with a partner who is infected with HPV.

There are vaccines that protect against HPVs, and these have been heavily recommended for boys and girls as young as 9 years of age up through their mid-20s in recent years. The vaccines only work to prevent an infection; they do not treat an existing infection, and the later in life that the HPV vaccines are administered, the less effective they are. However, there is growing concern that these vaccines can cause notable side effects and reactions, some of which are significant and life-altering.

If you want to be aggressive in preventing HPV, it is important to practice safe sex, or ideally, abstain until marriage.

Human T-Lymphotrophic Virus-1 (HTLV-1)

HTLV-1 is very rare in the United States; fewer than 1% of the population in the US is thought to be infected with the virus. Rates are higher in certain parts of Japan, the Caribbean, Africa, and parts of South America. HTLV-1 can cause other health problems, but often there are no symptoms. It is passed via unprotected sex and by sharing needles with infected people. HTLV-1 is linked with a type of cancer called adult T-cell leukemia/lymphoma (ATL). The risk associated with developing ATL can be as high as 5% after 20 years with no other symptoms. (20)

Merkel Cell Polyomavirus (MCV)

MCV was first discovered and described in 2008, and is thought to be associated with a very rare and aggressive skin cancer called Merkel cell carcinoma. (21) A large proportion of people are thought to have been exposed to this virus, likely early in life.

Ultimately, when it comes avoiding certain viruses with the intent to prevent cancer, cognizance is key. Many of these viruses are avoidable by not partaking in risky behaviors. Conversely, some are much more difficult to avoid. Optimizing immune system health is essential. However, if you are infected with a virus that is thought to elevate cancer risk, it is important to realize that you are certainly not guaranteed to develop cancer, you are just at an elevated risk. It is important to take other preventative measures to keep your "toxic bucket" from filling up any further.

Tip 6: Exercise Regularly

Exercise is something we all know that we should be doing, but many people fail to do it on a regular basis. Exercise comes with a legion of benefits, from cardiovascular improvements, to enhanced energy, to elevated mood. Many, however, do not realize that exercise reduces the risk of developing many cancers.

There are a variety of mechanisms behind exercise's cancer-preventing benefits. People who exercise tend to have a healthier weight, and people who maintain a healthy weight have a lower risk for developing cancer. (23) Exercise lowers inflammation in the body (24), and we know that heightened levels of inflammation are associated with a variety of diseases, including cancer. (25) People who exercise have lower insulin, and less insulin resistance, which reduces the risk of diabetes and cancer. (26) When you exercise, endorphins are released, which can stimulate the immune system and also play a potential role in preventing cancer.

Exercise also plays a key role in performing a vital bodily task; exercise floods the body with oxygen. When you elevate your heart rate and begin to breathe heavily, oxygen is dispersed throughout the body. According to Dr. Otto Warburg's research, cancer does not thrive in an oxygen-rich environment. It is likely that the increase in oxygen that is instigated by exercise creates an inhospitable environment for cancer cells. This reasoning is the basis for oxygenating treatments such as hyperbaric oxygen and ozone therapy.

Some studies have found a correlation between improving certain lifestyle factors, such as diet and physical activity, and the reduced risk of cancer. It is estimated that as many as 40% of cancer cases could be prevented simply by changing a few lifestyle factors, including exercise. (1) We have known this for some time now, but further research continues to affirm that exercise can play a big role in the prevention of cancer. A study of over 1.4 million participants published in 2016 found that regular physical activities reduce the risk for a number of cancers, including cancers of the colon, breast, endometrium, esophagus, liver, stomach, and kidney, as well as reducing the risk of myeloid leukemia. Other cancers that might also be prevented by regular exercise include cancers of the head and neck, rectum, bladder, and lung in both current and former smokers. (22)

This is an important finding, but there is another interesting fact that the authors concluded. The amount of exercise needed to reap the cancer-preventing benefits of physical activity was approximately 150 minutes a week of moderate exercise, or 75 minutes of vigorous exercise per week. A total of 150 minutes of weekly exercise equated to approximately 30 minutes a day, 5 days a week, walking at a 3 mph pace. Certainly, it takes a level of commitment to find the time to exercise. But the amount of exercise needed to reap the benefits of cancer prevention ultimately equates to spending half of what the average worker takes for lunch during the work week. The fact that such a little amount of time and effort on a regular basis can make such a profound difference in cancer prevention is a significant discovery.

Tip 7: Minimize Stress

When it comes to stress, anything that fills our "toxic bucket" could necessarily be considered a stressor on the body, but for our current discussion on stress, it is important that we focus on emotional stress and how it influences our health. Research over the past few decades has revealed that emotional stress instigates physical, biological responses in the body that can influence aspects of our health, including the development and progression of cancer.

As stated previously, Dr. Candace Pert was one of the pioneers in the field of exploring how our bodies are influenced by our emotions. In her book, *Molecules of Emotion*, she was one of the first to scientifically describe how emotions and emotional stress influence aspects of our health, such as digestion and our immune systems. While her work was met with some disbelief at the time, subsequent research has confirmed that stress can and does play a role in the progression of cancer. For example, we know that stress influences the progression of breast cancer. (27)

Whether or not stress can actually cause cancer, however, remains debated by many. There is evidence that striking life events, such as the sudden death of a loved one, can lead to the development of cancer. One meta-analysis concluded that there is "significant evidence for positive association between striking life events and primary breast cancer incidence in women." (28) Striking life events, of course, are certainly the kind of events that would create emotional stress in an individual. Should we not conclude, with relative certainty, that stress plays a prominent role in the development—and not just the progression—of cancer? I believe that we should.

Studies like these are similar to the work of Dr. Ryke Hamer. Dr. Harmer believed, and claimed to have significant evidence supporting the fact, that emotional stress set in motion by striking life events would ultimately lead to the development of cancer.

Dr. Hamer's theories remain controversial, and not surprisingly, mostly unacknowledged by conventional medicine. However, when we look at the cumulative research into emotions, stress, and cancer, we can confidently state that emotions play a notable role. If we are going to have a serious discussion about preventing and treating cancer, mitigating emotional stress and addressing previous life trauma must be included in that discussion. As you now know, this forms the basis for some of the treatments routinely used in integrative oncology.

Tip 8: Get Regular and Adequate Sleep

Getting quality sleep on a regular basis is a fundamental component of good health, but many do not realize that keeping normal, healthy sleeping patterns might play a role in preventing cancer.

An article published recently by the Harvard School of Public Health concluded that women regularly exposed to artificial light at night are at a greater risk for developing breast cancer. Women who worked the night shift were particularly at risk. The mechanism, they surmised, was due to the disruption of normal circadian rhythm patterns. (29)

Interestingly, the Harvard article was not the first to find a link between circadian rhythm disruption and cancer. A study published in 2014 came to similar conclusions; particularly, this study highlighted the importance of melatonin in breast cancer prevention. According to the researchers, melatonin reduces tumor growth and cell proliferation, inhibits angiogenesis, and prevents tumor development. (30) Other studies have also shown that melatonin has anti-cancer properties.

Melatonin is a hormone produced by the pineal gland. Melatonin helps regulate our normal 24-hour internal "clock," or circadian rhythm, and assists in promoting healthy sleep. Melatonin is produced in greater quantities in the dark, but its production can be disrupted in the presence of artificial light during the evening. This is why many sleep experts recommend keeping the room you sleep in completely dark. We can deduce that, given melatonin's anti-tumor activity, maintaining a healthy circadian rhythm and regularly getting adequate sleep are likely good cancer prevention mechanisms.

•————————————•

(1)   Song M, Giovannucci E. Preventable Incidence and Mortality of Carcinoma Associated With Lifestyle Factors Among White Adults in the United States." JAMA Oncology 2016; 2(9): 1154-61.

(2)   Jaslow R. "New car smell is toxic, study says: Which cars are worst?" CBS News, CBS Interactive, 15 Feb 2012, www.cbsnews.com/news/new-car-smell-is-toxic-study-says-which-cars-are-worst/. Accessed 14 Sept 2017.

(3) Kuhn DM, Ghannoum MA. Indoor mold, toxigenic fungi, and Stachybotrys chartarum: Infectious disease perspective. Clin Microbiol Rev 2003; 16(1): 144-72.

(4) Wickell J. "Do You Need to Inspect a Home for Radan Gas?" The Balance, www.thebalance.com/facts-about-radon-gas-testing-1797839. Accessed 14 Sept 2017.

(5) "How air pollution can cause cancer." Cancer Research UK, 10 July 2017, www.cancerresearchuk.org/about-cancer/causes-of-cancer/air-pollution-radon-gas-and-cancer/how-air-pollution-can-cause-cancer. Accessed 14 Sept 2017.

(6) "World Health Organization: Outdoor Air Pollution Causes Cancer." American Cancer Society, www.cancer.org/latest-news/world-health-organization-outdoor-air-pollution-causes-cancer.html. Accessed 14 Sept 2017.

(7) López-Carrillo L, Hernandez-Ramirez RU, Calafat AM, et al. Exposure to phthalates and breast cancer risk in northern Mexico. Environ Health Perspect 2010; 118(4): 539-44.

(8) "Lotion ingredient paraben may be more potent carcinogen than thought." Berkeley News, 29 Oct 2015, news.berkeley.edu/2015/10/27/lotion-ingredient-paraben-may-be-more-potent-carcinogen-than-thought/. Accessed 15 Sept 2017.

(9) "Talcum Powder and Cancer." American Cancer Society, www.cancer.org/cancer/cancer-causes/talcum-powder-and-cancer.html. Accessed 15 Sept 2017.

(10) Betts KS. New thinking on flame retardants. Environ Health Perspect 2008; 116(5): A210-13.

(11) "Cancer-linked Flame Retardants Eased Out of Furniture in 2014." Scientific American, www.scientificamerican.com/article/cancer-linked-flame/. Accessed 15 Sept. 2017.

(12) "Dry Cleaning Chemical 'Likely' Causes Cancer." WebMD, 9 Feb. 2010, www.webmd.com/cancer/news/20100209/dry-cleaning-chemical-likely-causes-cancer#1. Accessed 15 Sept 2017.

(13) "Chlorinated water - Canadian Cancer Society." www.cancer.ca/en/prevention-and-screening/be-aware/harmful-substances-and-environmental-risks/chlorinated-water/?region=on. Accessed 15 Sept 2017.

(14) "Skin Deep® Cosmetics Database | EWG." Skin Deep Home Comments, www.ewg.org/skindeep/#.WbwW3bRH2Rs. Accessed 15 Sept 2017.

(15) "Obesity and Cancer." National Cancer Institute, www.cancer.gov/about-cancer/causes-prevention/risk/obesity/obesity-fact-sheet. Accessed 15 Sept 2017.

(16) "Type 2 Diabetes: The Basics." WebMD, www.webmd.com/diabetes/type-2-diabetes-guide/type-2-diabetes#1. Accessed 15 Sept 2017.

(17) "Why Does Diabetes Raise Cancer Risk?" WebMD, www.webmd.com/diabetes/news/20100616/why-does-diabetes-increase-cancer-risk. Accessed 15 Sept 2017.

(18) "Low LDL Cholesterol is Related to Cholesterol Risk." American College of Cardiology, http://www.acc.org/about-acc/press-releases/2012/03/25/15/15/ldl_cancer. Accessed 15 Sept 2017.

(19) "Development of Modern Knowledge about Cancer Causes." American Cancer Society, https://www.cancer.org/cancer/cancer-basics/history-of-cancer/modern-knowledge-and-cancer-causes.html. Accessed 26 July 2017.

(20) "Viruses that can lead to cancer." American Cancer Society, www.cancer.org/cancer/cancer-causes/infectious-agents/infections-that-can-lead-to-cancer/viruses.html. Accessed 27 Sept 2017.

(21) Malaria and some polyomaviruses (SV40, BK, JC, and Merkel cell viruses). Lyon, IARC Press, 2012.

(22) "Exercise Linked With Lower Risk of 13 Types of Cancer." American Cancer Society, www.cancer.org/latest-news/exercise-linked-with-lower-risk-of-13-types-of-cancer.html. Accessed 28 Sept 2017.

(23) Vainio H, Kaaka R, Bianchini F. Weight control and physical activity in cancer prevention: international evaluation of the evidence. Eur J Cancer Prev 2002; 11 Suppl: S94-100.

(24) Woods, Jeffery A, et al. "Exercise, Inflammation and Aging." Aging and Disease, vol. 3, no. 1, 29 Oct. 2011, pp. 130–40.

(25) Coussens LM, Werb Z. Inflammation and cancer. Nature 2002; 420(6917): 860-7.

(26) Borghouts LB, Keizer HA. Exercise and insulin sensitivity: a review. Int J Sports Med 2000; 21(1): 1-12.

(27) Moreno-Smith M, Lutgendorf SK, Sood AK. Impact of stress on cancer metastasis. Future Oncol 2010; 6(12): 1863-81.

(28) Lin Y, Wang C, Zhong Y, et al. Striking life events associated with primary breast cancer susceptibility in women: a meta-analysis study. J Exp Clin Cancer Res 2013; 32(1): 53.

(29) James P, Bertrand KA, Hart JE, et al. Outdoor light and night and breast cancer incidence in the nurses' health study II. Environ Health Perspect 2017; 125(8): 087010.

(30) Zamfir Chiru AA, Popescu CR, Gheorghe DC. Melatonin and cancer. J Med Life 2014; 7(3): 373-4.

APPENDIX A

Food List

Focus on These Foods:

Vegetables

Asparagus

Beets

Bell peppers

Bok choy

Broccoli

Brussels sprouts

Cabbage

Carrots

Cauliflower

Celery

Collard greens

Cucumbers

Eggplant

Green beans

Kale

Leeks

Lettuce

Mustard greens

Okra

Onions

Parsley

Pumpkin

Romaine

Spinach

Squash

Sweet potatoes

Swiss chard

Turnip greens

Watercress

Zucchini

<u>Fruits</u>

Apples
Apricots
Avocados
Bananas
Blackberries
Blueberries
Cantaloupe
Cranberries
Dates
Figs
Grapefruit

Grapes
Honeydew melon
Kiwi
Lemons
Limes
Mangoes
Nectarines
Olives
Oranges
Papayas
Peaches

Pears
Pineapples
Plantains
Plums
Raisins
Raspberries
Strawberries
Tangerines
Tomatoes
Watermelon

<u>Grains</u>

Amaranth
Barley
Buckwheat
Hominy

Kamut
Oats
Quinoa
Spelt

Tapioca
Wheat (sprouted or
ancient only)

<u>Herbs and Spices</u>

Basil
Black pepper
Chili pepper
Cilantro seeds
Cinnamon
Cloves
Cumin

Dill
Fennel
Garlic
Ginger
Mustard seeds
Oregano
Parsley

Peppermint
Rosemary
Sage
Thyme
Turmeric

Legumes

Black-eyed peas
Hummus
Lentils
Miso
Okra

Nuts & Seeds

Almonds
Flaxseeds
Hazelnuts
Macadamia nuts
Pecans
Walnuts

Oils

Coconut oil
Flax oil
Olive oil

●————————————————————●

Limit These Foods:

Dairy
Cheese
Eggs
Yogurt

Legumes
Black beans
Fava beans
Lima beans
Navy beans
Refried beans
Split peas
Tofu

Sweeteners
Honey
Maple syrup
Molasses

Meats/Animal Protein
Beef
Bison
Chicken
Lamb
Salmon
Tuna

Nuts & Seeds
Cashews
Chia seeds
Pistachios
Pumpkin seeds
Sesame seeds

Vegetables
Corn
Peas
White potatoes

Avoid These Foods:

Grains

White flour
Gluten (except ancient grains)
Teff

Legumes

Peanuts
Soybeans

Meats/Animal Protein

Bacon
Catfish
Lobster
Mussels
Oysters
Pork
Shrimp

Oils

Hydrogenated oils
Trans fats

Sweeteners

Aspartame
Sucralose
Sugar

Vegetables

Mushrooms

Made in the USA
Middletown, DE
21 May 2019